Homeopathy

Homeopathy

An Illusion of Effectiveness

Dinesh Kumar Jain BSc, MBBS, MD

Formerly – Professor and Head
Pharmacology Department
Bundelkhand Medical College Sagar, India

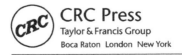

CRC Press is an imprint of the
Taylor & Francis Group, an **informa** business

First edition published 2022
by CRC Press
6000 Broken Sound Parkway NW, Suite 300, Boca Raton, FL 33487-2742

and by CRC Press
4 Park Square, Milton Park, Abingdon, Oxon, OX14 4RN

CRC Press is an imprint of Taylor & Francis Group, LLC

© 2022 Dinesh Kumar Jain

Reasonable efforts have been made to publish reliable data and information, but the author and publisher cannot assume responsibility for the validity of all materials or the consequences of their use. The authors and publishers have attempted to trace the copyright holders of all material reproduced in this publication and apologize to copyright holders if permission to publish in this form has not been obtained. If any copyright material has not been acknowledged please write and let us know so we may rectify in any future reprint.

Except as permitted under U.S. Copyright Law, no part of this book may be reprinted, reproduced, transmitted, or utilized in any form by any electronic, mechanical, or other means, now known or hereafter invented, including photocopying, microfilming, and recording, or in any information storage or retrieval system, without written permission from the publishers.

For permission to photocopy or use material electronically from this work, access www.copyright.com or contact the Copyright Clearance Center, Inc. (CCC), 222 Rosewood Drive, Danvers, MA 01923, 978-750-8400. For works that are not available on CCC please contact mpkbookspermissions@tandf.co.uk

Trademark notice: Product or corporate names may be trademarks or registered trademarks and are used only for identification and explanation without intent to infringe.

Library of Congress Cataloging-in-Publication Data

Names: Jain, Dinesh Kumar, author.
Title: Homeopathy : an illusion of effectiveness / Dinesh Kumar Jain,
   B.Sc., M.B.B.S., M.D., Formerly - Professor and Head, Pharmacology
   Department, Bundelkhand Medical College Sagar, India.
Description: First edition. | Boca Raton : Taylor and Francis, 2022. |
   Includes bibliographical references and index.
Identifiers: LCCN 2021057267 (print) | LCCN 2021057268 (ebook) | ISBN
   9781032133133 (hardback) | ISBN 9781032113227 (paperback) | ISBN
   9781003228622 (ebook)
Subjects: LCSH: Homeopathy.
Classification: LCC RX71 .J35 2022 (print) | LCC RX71 (ebook) | DDC
   615.5/32--dc23
LC record available at https://lccn.loc.gov/2021057267
LC ebook record available at https://lccn.loc.gov/2021057268

ISBN: 978-1-032-13313-3 (hbk)
ISBN: 978-1-032-11322-7 (pbk)
ISBN: 978-1-003-22862-2 (ebk)

DOI: 10.1201/9781003228622

Typeset in Palatino
by KnowledgeWorks Global Ltd.

Contents

Preface ix
About the author xi
Introduction xiii

Chapter 1   Like cures like 1

Chapter 2   Dilution increases potency 5

Chapter 3   Criticism of allopathy 9

Chapter 4   Knowledge regarding diseases 13

Chapter 5   Nomenclature of diseases 15

Chapter 6   Cures means removal of symptoms 17

Chapter 7   External factors for diseases 19

Chapter 8   Rejection of pathological investigations 23

Chapter 9   Mechanism of cure 25

Chapter 10   Interaction of diseases 29

Chapter 11   Causes of chronic diseases 33

Chapter 12   Change the drug treatment 35

Chapter 13   Only homeopathy is best 37

Chapter 14   Curative power of medicine 39

v

Chapter 15 Displacement of pathological symptoms 45

Chapter 16 Mercuric chloride and syphilis 51

Chapter 17 Effect of opium 55

Chapter 18 Manic episode 59

Chapter 19 Scarlet fever and belladonna 63

Chapter 20 Grinding gives power and color 67

Chapter 21 Treatment of cholera 71

Chapter 22 Psora 75

Chapter 23 Development of psora 79

Chapter 24 Skin diseases 83

Chapter 25 Wart and localized treatment 87

Chapter 26 Psychiatric symptoms 91

Chapter 27 Dynamization 95

Chapter 28 Fever, injection, and vaccination 99

Chapter 29 Suffering with two dissimilar diseases 101

Chapter 30 Tuberculosis 109

Chapter 31 One disease protects from another disease 113

Chapter 32 Therapeutic effectiveness 117

Chapter 33 Bright's disease and syphilis 127

Chapter 34 Fistula in ano 131

Chapter 35 No organ can make the body sick 133

Chapter 36 Bacteria are harmless 135

Contents *vii*

Chapter 37 Hahnemann opposed old school of medicine...................143

Chapter 38 Termination of acute and chronic disease 145

Chapter 39 Syphilis causes termination of life.....................................149

Chapter 40 Treatment of syphilis 155

Chapter 41 Sycosis...163

Chapter 42 Venereal diseases 165

Chapter 43 Chancroid and chancre 173

Chapter 44 Allopathic drugs suppress symptoms 175

Chapter 45 Fig-wart diseases and gonorrhea.......................................179

Chapter 46 Suppressed manifestations must come back......................187

Chapter 47 Psora and spiritualism 191

Chapter 48 St. Anthony's fire and leprosy 195

Chapter 49 Pathogenesis of psora 199

Chapter 50 Awakening of internal psora..203

Chapter 51 Suppression of itch and tinea capitis 207

Chapter 52 Epilepsy and exanthema...213

Chapter 53 Confusion 219

Chapter 54 Repetition of dose and medicine 221

Chapter 55 Hahnemann accepted failure..227

Chapter 56 Research on homeopathy..239

Chapter 57 Conclusion 255

Index 261

Preface

Samuel Hahnemann of Germany (1755–1843) developed a new system of therapeutics: homeopathy. Worldwide, over 250–300 million people are using homeopathy today.

Principles of homeopathy are not according to principles of basic medical science. Concepts of basic medical science oppose concepts of homeopathy. WHO stated that "inappropriate use of traditional medicines or practices can have negative or dangerous effects".

Modern medical science is based on experiments, lab studies, evidence-based observations, animal studies, clinical trials, continuous and dedicated efforts of scientists, and knowledge of all branches of science. In contrast, homeopathy is based on religious and philosophical beliefs of culture and hypothetical unscientific observations.

Hahnemann arrived at wrong conclusions on the basis of faulty analysis due to lack of knowledge. There was no knowledge of human physiology, pathology, pathogenesis, or investigations in Hahnemann's time, which is why he had limitations. He formulated unscientific and illogical hypotheses.

Hahnemann's observations, analysis, and conclusions which were homeopathy's basis of origin have been examined in this work.

I studied in detail the manufacturing process of homeopathic medicines. I tried to cover all the pharmacological aspects of these drugs. The study and experiments were not done as prescribed by modern medical science. Pharmacological data of these drugs are not available. There is no pharmacokinetic or pharmacodynamic study of homeopathic remedies. Hahnemann mentioned that diseases had been cured by homeopathic drugs. After studying the normal course of such diseases, it has been found that these diseases had been cured spontaneously. Spontaneously curable diseases had given the wrong impression to Hahnemann that such diseases had been treated by highly diluting homeopathic drugs.

I also studied mistakes made by Hahnemann during his research and puzzled over why he commited these mistakes. Today we have vast and developed medical knowledge. Whatever has been said in favor of homeopathy, we have analyzed in context of present medical knowledge and found them to be absolutely wrong. And in this way, in this work it has been concluded that principles of homeopathy are inaccurate, useless, and homeopathic drugs have no therapeutic utility.

I am greatly indebted to Mr. Stephen M. Zollo, senior editor, CRC Press/Taylor & Francis Group, who showed confidence in my work and inspired me to do this work efficiently. His voracious appetite for knowledge, an infectious enthusiasm for publication, a keen appreciation for analytical rigor, and a genuine affinity for creation have had a significant impact on the final structure of this text. Thanks to Ms. Laura Piedrahita for her valuable suggestions in preparation of the manuscript. Also thanks to Ms. Manisha Singh Pundir for her excellent and marvellous copyediting and typesetting work for turning my manuscript into printable pages. And I am extremely grateful to Taylor & Francis Group for publishing my work.

Dinesh Kumar Jain

About the author

Dinesh Kumar Jain, BSc, MBBS, MD (Pharmacology), has worked as a professor of pharmacology in Bundelkhand Medical College, Sagar, India. He is an expert pharmacologist, renowned medical teacher, psychological counselor, poet, and social reformer. He has been nominated as best teacher by medical students, and is known for his lively lectures. He earned degrees in psychological counseling, family education, and religion. He experienced extreme hardship and endless struggle in his life due to the problematic, fatuous, suffocating, and unhealthy traditions and social norms of Indian society. This painful journey motivated him to reform Indian society.

He wrote a book on the Indian marriage system (published in 1997, BHARAT ME VIVAH EK NASUR – Marriage system in India, a cancer). The Indian system of arranged marriage is actually damaging Indian society. Most of the problems in Indian society are the result of the prevalent marriage system.

He formed an NGO AVEKSHA for the purpose of social reform.

Dr. Jain has also written weekly columns in newspapers, *Dainik Bhaskar, Gwalior, MP* and *Dainik Jagran, Agra, UP*, as a psychological counselor to solve personal, psychological, and social problems. He also worked as an honorary psychological counselor.

He has published many research papers in national and international journals. Main subjects of his research work are (a) to study therapeutic effectiveness of Ayurveda, homeopathy, yoga and pranayam and questioning their therapeutic efficacy, (b) analysis of alloxan-induced diabetic model, (c) explanation of mechanism of action of class 1 antiarrhythmic drugs and the effect of potassium on the heart using mathematical models and mathematical calculations. His work has been published in the *World Journal of Pharmaceutical Research, Indian Journal of Pharmacology, Journal of Pharmacovigilance and Drug Safety, International Journal of Basic and Clinical Pharmacology.*

Dr. Jain's aim in life is to remove social problems and unscientific concepts from Indian society. He has accomplished this by giving lectures, providing scientific facts, and writing books and research papers. He fights to improve the social system of India and eliminate social evils, unhealthy traditions, and unscientific values.

Introduction

One of the most important aims of human life is to develop human potential and do creative work for the welfare of society and the new generation. Creation of knowledge is a continuous process. History of knowledge is closely associated with the history of human beings. Continuous efforts of civilizations are responsible for continuous accumulation of knowledge. In earlier times, there was very limited knowledge. Today, we have vast knowledge which is the sum of the creative efforts of thousands of years by millions of humans. On the basis of this knowledge, new concepts and new thoughts can be deduced.

New generations have greater knowledge than older generations, that's why they can make better decisions than older generations, and they can also change decisions and assumptions of old generations. Beliefs, traditions, and concepts of our forefathers should be changed if they are found unsuitable in the context of present evolved knowledge.

"The great Greek physician Hippocrates (460–377 B.C.) has been called the father of modern medicine. He denied the intervention of deities and demons in the development of disease" (Coleman, 1976, p. 27).

Before Hippocrates, it was presumed that all diseases were due to supernatural influences. Hippocrates provided revolutionary concepts which made him responsible for the development of modern medical science. Not only Hippocrates but many intellectuals also contributed to the development of present knowledge. Progressive ideas and concepts could be determined only after verification by present evolved knowledge. If a concept or a theory cannot be verified by experiments, analysis, and arguments, then this concept or theory should be discarded.

Samuel Hahnemann of Germany (1755–1843) developed a new system of therapeutics, homeopathy. Today around the world, more than 250 million–300 million people and at least 60–70 countries use homeopathy.

> Currently homeopathy has been integrated into the national health care systems of many countries, including India, Mexico, Pakistan, Sri Lanka, and the

xiii

> United Kingdom. In the World Health Organization report about alternative medicine that was published in 2001, we noticed that homeopathy is regulated in 45 countries (Asia 7, Africa 7, America 9, Australia 2 and Europe 20). (Mazaherinezhad, 2004)

According to one study of prevalence of homeopathy use by the general population worldwide over 12 months, this review summarizes results from surveys conducted in eleven countries (the USA, the UK, Australia, Israel, Canada, Switzerland, Norway, Germany, South Korea, Japan, and Singapore). Rate of prevalence of homeopathy use by the general population ranged from .2 to 9.8% in different review surveys (Relton et al., 2017). If we take the prevalence of homeopathy use, 5% as an average, then it can be estimated that 300 million–350 million people in the world use homeopathy.

"India leads in terms of number of people using homeopathy, with 100 million people depending solely on homeopathy for their medical care" (Mazaherinezhad, 2004, as cited in Prasad, 2007). Six million people in the UK, 100 million EU citizens use homeopathy (Mazaherinezhad, 2004).

> Homeopathy reached its peak of popularity in the early 1900s. Today there is a resurgence in the popularity of this old medical method ...Today there are about 3000 recognized practitioners in the U.S. whose practice is mostly homeopathic ... In France 16% of the population uses homeopathic drug products on a regular basis and 90% of the pharmacies sell homeopathic drug products. In England 45% of conventional physicians refer patients to homeopathic practitioners and this number is increasing at an annual rate of 39% ... In Russia at least 20% of the medical care is homeopathic. Homeopathy has a strong following in Belgium, Germany, Netherlands, Italy and South America. Homeopathy traditionally has had a strong following in poorer countries. For example, India has 100,000 prescribers of homeopathic medicine. (Marderosian et al., 2000, p. 1771)

This indicates homeopathy is becoming popular throughout the world. But rules of homeopathy and concepts of modern medical science are contradictory to each other. Either modern medical science or homeopathy is correct. If we are saying that both are correct, this indicates our

Introduction

xv

inefficiency and incapabilities to reach a definite conclusion. If homeopathy is wrong and it is popular with the common man, then we, scientific persons, are committing crimes against humanity and science.

In this work, I have analyzed the principles of homeopathy made by Hahnemann. The analysis has been done in the context of present knowledge of medical science.

If homeopathy is accurate, then costly modern allopathy should be replaced by homeopathy. If homeopathy is wrong and treatment of diseases is not possible by homeopathy, then it should not be recommended and it is no use to spend money and time on homeopathy.

I have studied deep and reached this conclusion that homeopathy is absolutely wrong. Principles of homeopathy are baseless and homeopathic drugs have no therapeutic effect.

Rich and resourceful populations first take modern medical therapy. In incurable and chronic diseases, they take homeopathic medicine just for change. They never prefer homeopathy as a first-line treatment. Homeopathy always remains the second alternative method for these rich and educated people. Such illogical use establishes homeopathy unnecessarily. Poor and uneducated populations prefer homeopathy because it is cheaper and then they suffer the most. Patients with tuberculosis, cancer, malaria, or typhoid die in these families because they were taking homeopathic medicines for these ailments. There are many glaucomatous blind members in these families because they are not going for eye surgery but taking homeopathic drugs. Tuberculosis, leprosy, and malaria are increasing day by day because people are not completing the courses of modern allopathic drugs but instead shift toward homeopathy. Then drugs become resistant. Homeopathy is a hobby or fashion for richer and resourceful persons but this is a death door for poor and uneducated people. Who will be responsible for this crime? Are national and international scientific communities ready to take responsibility for such an offense?

The aim of my work is to find the truth and protect poor and uneducated people from dangerous consequences of homeopathy because people ignore advantageous medical science. Also, the aim of my work is to remove illogical and wrong concepts from science and help in the evolution of knowledge.

This book will be highly useful to the medical fraternity as well as the nonmedical fraternity, in dispelling several myths associated with homeopathy. It will help medical personnel to develop a rational approach toward homeopathy, based on scientific facts and will ultimately promote evidence-based medicine. After reading this book, readers will gain more knowledge about different medical systems of medicine and understand modern medical science. A common man will change his attitude. He will

xvi *Introduction*

develop a scientific temperament. Societies can use money and infrastructure for the implementation of therapeutically useful systems rather than unnecessary wastage of resources in implementation of useless therapeutic systems.

Dinesh Kumar Jain

References

Coleman, J. (1976). *Abnormal psychology and modern life*. Bombay, India: Taraporewala and Sons.

Marderosian, A. H. D., Krantz, A. M., & Riedlinger, J. E. (2000). Complementary & alternative medical health care. In A. R. Gennaro (Ed.), *Remington: The science and practice of pharmacy* (20th ed., Vol. 2, pp. 1762–1779). Philadelphia, PA: Lippincott, Williams & Wilkins.

Mazaherinezhad, A. (2004). Homeopathy use around the world. *Iranian Journal of Pharmaceutical Research*, 3(Supplement 2), 11–11. Supplement 2.

Prasad, R. (2007). Homeopathy booming in India. *Lancet*, 370, 1679–1680

Relton, C., Cooper, K., Petter, V. P., Fibert, P., & Thomas, K. (2017). Prevalence of homeopathy use by the general population worldwide: A systematic review. *Homeopathy*, 106(2), 69–78. doi: 10.1016/j.homp.2017.03.002.

chapter one

Like cures like

Basic concept of homeopathy – one

There are two important principles of homeopathy. First, "like cures like", which means treatment of a disease by the use of a small amount of drug that produces symptoms in healthy persons similar to those of the disease being treated.

Argument

There are two important principles of homeopathy. First, "like cures like", which means if the symptoms of disease can be reproduced in the healthy body by a drug, then that drug is effective in that disease.

> Similar symptoms in the remedy remove similar symptoms of the disease. The eternal, universal law of Nature, that every disease is destroyed and cured through the similar artificial disease which the appropriate remedy has the tendency to excite, rests on the following proposition: that only one disease can exist in the body at any one time. (Bennett & Brown, 2008, p. 16)

Second important principle of homeopathy is, "Dilution potentiates the action of drugs. Homeopathy outlines the therapy for various ailments with drugs in very high dilutions" (Satoskar et al., 2015, p. 1). "Lower concentration of a remedy (properly diluted and shaken vigorously {succussed}), the greater the effectiveness" (Marderosian et al., 2000, p. 1770). According to Hahnemann, the effect of drugs is potentiated by dilution even to the extent that an effective dose may not contain a single molecule of drug. Regarding dilution, "Thirtieth potency (1 in 10^{30}), recommended by Hahnemann, provided a solution in which there would be one molecule of drug in a volume of a sphere of literally astronomical circumference" (Bennett & Brown, 2008, p. 16).

Both of these principles of homeopathy were analyzed and found that the conclusion drawn by Hahnemann was wrong. "Hahnemann's first principle was a generalization based on the fact that a large dose of cinchona bark induced in him a malarial paroxysm. The reason for this

DOI: 10.1201/9781003228622-1

occurrence being that he had previously suffered from malaria and the gastric irritation excited the paroxysm" (Modell et al., 1976, p. 9).

Hahnemann could not understand the fact that his suffering with malaria and gastric irritation by cinchona bark was responsible for his recurrence of paroxysm. The cinchona bark contains quinine alkaloid. This alkaloid has antimalarial action. "In malarial fever, quinine has a direct action on the organism causing the disease and suppresses the elevated body temperature. Quinine may exercise a true antipyretic action. The effect of quinine on normal body temperature is negligible" (Krantz & Carr, 1965, p. 158). "Quinine has analgesic and antipyretic action and a definite lowering of body temperature occurs in fever from any cause. For this reason quinine has been used in many symptomatic remedies" (Dipalma, 1965, p. 1388).

> Rigors or chills are common at the onset of various febrile disorders and may occur at regular or irregular intervals. The cardinal feature of rigor is shivering. Chills and rigors may **be produced and perpetuated by intermittent administration of an effective antipyretic agent.** This may cause a sharp depression of a raised temperature in a febrile state which precipitates involuntary muscular contraction. (Hart, 1985b, p. 737)

"Initially rigors also occur in acute gastrointestinal disorder" (French, 1945, p. 744).

There is always a possibility of relapse of malaria. Relapses of malaria occur when malarial parasites persisting in the liver, reenter the bloodstream, and patients should be followed for one month to detect the infection (Plorde, 1983, pp. 1190–1192). The form of malarial parasite that persists in the liver is not destroyed by quinine present in cinchona bark. It was observed, "Malaria may remain latent for many years. Reappearance is brought about by cold, general depression of health or through some intercurrent malady" (Hart, 1985a, p. 285).

The main constituent of cinchona bark is quinine. "Oral administration of quinine often results in nausea, vomiting and epigastric pain" (Satoskar & Bhandarkar, 1988, p. 655).

By these observations we can conclude the following:

1. Quinine is the main component of cinchona bark, which is effective against malarial fever. Effect of quinine on normal body temperature is negligible.
2. Hahnemann had suffered from malaria. Just after this, he took cinchona bark and got malarial paroxysm. The cause of this incidence

Chapter one: Like cures like   3

can be explained as: (a) within one month of malarial attack, the chance of malaria relapse is very high. Relapse may occur by acute gastrointestinal problem or any intercurrent malady. Hahnemann had taken cinchona after symptomatic cure of malaria. Gastrointestinal problems created by cinchona could be responsible for recurrence of malarial paroxysm. Normal body temperature is not altered and malarial paroxysm does not occur in a normal healthy person after taking cinchona. (b) Second explanation can also be given for recurrence of malarial paroxysm. At the time of Hahnemann, the actual cause of malaria was not known. Ronald Ross discovered the transmission of malaria by anopheline mosquitoes in 1897 and also discovered malarial parasites, and diagnosis of malaria depends on identification of the parasite in the blood (Park, 1997, pp. 188–193). The paroxysm of fever with chill, which Hahnemann suffered after taking cinchona, might not be malaria, because at that time the cause of malaria was not known. So confirmation of malaria was not possible by demonstration of malarial parasites in blood. There are so many causes of fever with chills. It might be possible that Hahnemann had suffered from other diseases having symptoms of fever with chill. It was just coincidence that at that time he took cinchona and he wrongly concluded that this paroxysm was of malaria and due to cinchona.

If the principle of homeopathy is true, then quinine should produce rigor in a healthy body. But studies say that quinine does not produce rigor. If Hahnemann is true, then quinine should produce rigors in the healthy body because quinine is effective in malaria, which is characterized by rigors with fever. I will write again that in medical science, conclusions cannot be drawn by single observation or observation in a few persons. Those doctors who believe in single observation or observation in a few persons and draw conclusions on this basis only don't know anything regarding medical science. During single observation or observation in single or few persons, there are various factors which may influence the observation and thus give wrong conclusions.

Hahnemann and his followers made this mistake. In therapeutics, controlled study and experiments on many patients, decided with the rules of statistics, should be done to draw the right conclusion.

References

Bennett, P. N., & Brown, M. J. (2008). *Clinical pharmacology* (10th ed.). Edinburgh, United Kingdom: Churchill Livingstone.

Dipalma, R. J. (1965). Chemotherapy of protozoan infections: Malaria. In J. R. Dipalma (Ed.), *Drill's pharmacology in medicine* (3rd ed., pp. 1376–1391). New York, NY: McGraw Hill Book Company.

French, H. (1945). *An index of differential diagnosis of main symptoms* (6th ed.). Bristol, United Kingdom: John Wright.

Hart, F. D. (1985a). Fever prolonged (prolonged pyrexia). In F.D. Hart (Ed.), *French's index of differential diagnosis* (12th ed., pp. 275–288). London, United Kingdom: Wright.

Hart, F. D. (1985b). Rigors or chills. In F. D. Hart (Ed.), *French's index of differential diagnosis* (12th ed., pp. 737–740). London, United Kingdom: Wright.

Krantz, J. C., & Carr, C. J. (1965). *The pharmacological principles of medical practice* (Indian 6th ed.). Baltimore, MD: Williams and Wilkins Company.

Marderosian, A. H. D., Krantz, A. M., & Riedlinger, J. E. (2000). Complementary and alternative medical health care. In A. R. Gennaro (Ed.), *Remington: The science and practice of pharmacy* (20th ed., Vol. 2, pp. 1762–1779). Philadelphia, PA: Lippincott Williams and Wilkins.

Modell, W., Schield, H., & Wilson, A. (1976). *Applied pharmacology* (American ed.). Toronto: W.B. Saunders Company.

Park, K. (1997). *Park's textbook of preventive and social medicine* (15th ed.). Jabalpur, India: Banarsidas Bhanot Publisher.

Plorde, J. J. (1983). Malaria. In R. G. Petersdorf, R. D. Adams, E. Braunwald, K. J. Isselbacher, J. B. Martin, & J. D. Wilson (Eds.), *Harrison's principle of internal medicine* (10th ed., pp. 1187–1193). New Delhi, India: McGraw Hill.

Satoskar, R. S. & Bhandarkar, S. D. (1988). *Pharmacology and pharmacotherapeutics* (11th ed.). Mumbai, India: Elsevier and Popular Prakashan.

Satoskar, R. S., Rege, N. N., & Bhandarkar, S. D. (2015). *Pharmacology and pharmacotherapeutics* (24th ed.). Mumbai, India: Elsevier and Popular Prakashan.

chapter two

Dilution increases potency

Basic concept of homeopathy – two

Second important principle of homeopathy is dilution and trituration potentiates the potency of a drug.

Argument

Second important principle of homeopathy is, "Dilution potentiates the potency". Hahnemann derived this principle by the following observation and experiment. Hahnemann found that "Trituration of mercury increased its pharmacological effect" (Modell et al., 1976, p. 9). He observed that potency of mercury increased after dilution and trituration. Later on this conclusion was analyzed and it was found that increased potency of mercury was not due to dilute and triturated mercury. "This increased effect was due to oxidation of mercury, first to mercurous and later to mercuric oxide" (Modell et al., 1976, p. 9). The potentiated effect that Hahnemann observed was due to mercuric oxide. This second important principle of homeopathy again was due to wrong generalization of wrong observation.

Today it is also known that "Elemental mercury cannot react with biologically important molecules. When ingested or taken orally, it occurs as large globular particles in the G.I.T. and is absorbed very poorly. The soluble inorganic mercuric salts gain access to the circulation when taken orally" (Klaassen, 1980, p. 1623). It has also been found that "Mercury is easily converted into the form of a dull grey powder when triturated with sugar, chalk or lard. The process is known as deadening. Grey powder contains 33% of mercury and a portion of the mercury is converted into mercuric oxide which produces a poisonous action on the system" (Modi, 1975, p. 545). "Cases are recorded where individuals have swallowed a pound or two of the liquid metal (perfectly pure) without any harmful effect" (Modi, 1975, p. 551).

> "The salts of mercury and silver dissolved in water have been used as antiseptic solutions for many years. Today these substances have to a large extent been replaced by less toxic organic chemicals. Solutions of mercuric chloride are useful in

DOI: 10.1201/9781003228622-2

disinfecting materials. Aqueous solutions of 1:100 to 1:10000 dilutions are generally employed" (Krantz & Carr, 1965, p. 551).

Now it is very clear that mercury in pure form is an inert substance when given orally but mercuric compounds obtained after trituration of mercury are highly potent and effective in more dilutions. Now it can be said that it was not dilution and trituration that increased potency of mercury; it was actually conversion of mercury into mercuric oxide, which was responsible for increased potency.

Now we are taking another parameter. If dilution increases potency, then dilute drug should have stronger action than concentrated drug. Observations do not prove this statement.

Observations in patients prove that concentrated drugs have stronger and more potent action than dilute drugs. Few examples are being given.

Methylmercury in blood produces various manifestations. Blood concentration of 0.1–0.5 µg/ml produces no ataxia, no visual defect, no hearing defect and no death. Blood concentration of 1–2 µg/ml of methyl mercury causes ataxia in 47% persons, visual defect in 53% cases, hearing defect in 5% cases and no death; while blood concentration of 4–5 µg/ml produces ataxia in 100% cases, visual defect in 83% cases, hearing defect in 66% cases and death in 28% cases. (Klaassen, 1980, p. 1624)

Behavior and physiological effects of ethanol in humans associated with increasing blood ethanol concentration also prove that the Hahnemann principle of dilution is wrong. When ethanol concentration of blood is increased, toxic effects are also increased, while Hahnemann said dilution increased potency of a drug:

"Blood concentration of alcohol and effect

1. <50 mg/dl causes euphoria, sedation, high sociability, euphoria
2. 50–100 mg/dl causes increased reaction time, lack of concentration, altered gait
3. 100–200 mg/dl causes impaired motor function, ataxia, slurred speech
4. 200–300 mg/dl causes emesis, stupor, no response to sensory stimuli
5. 300–400 mg/dl causes coma
6. Greater than 400 mg/dl causes respiratory depression and death" (Srivastav, 2016, p. 485).

Chapter two: Dilution increases potency 7

"Plasma concentration of Lithium in mania should range from 0.9 to 1.4 mEq/L. Concentration higher than 1.5 mEq/L is associated with an increased incidence of side effects, while those about 2 mEq/L may result in serious toxicity" (Ward & Azzaro, 1997, p. 394).

Now it is clear that dilution does not increase potency.

> From 1829 onward Hahnemann recommended the administration of all drugs at the thirtieth potency which corresponds to a concentration of 1 part in 10^{60} parts (10 to the power of 60). This works out at a content of 1 molecule of drug in a sphere with a circumference equal to the orbit of Neptune. (Modell et al., 1976, p. 9)

The distance between Neptune and the Sun is 4496.6×10^6 kilometers. This is the radius of the sphere produced by Neptune around the sun. The volume of this sphere will be $4/3\ \pi r^3$. It will be equal to

$$= 4/3\ \pi \times r \times r \times r$$

$$= 4/3 \times 22/7 \times 4496.6 \times 4496.6 \times 4496.6 \times 10^6 \times 10^6 \times 10^6$$

$$= 363 \times 10^{27} \text{ cubic km approximately}$$

We can conclude that a container of 70,000 lacs kilometer length, 70,000 lacs kilometer width, and 70,000 lacs kilometer height, which is filled with homeopathic drug of 30th potency will contain only one molecule of homeopathic drug.

We can also explain in another way. If we give homeopathic drugs to a patient in that amount which is equal to the water contained in all the rivers and oceans on the earth will not contain any molecule of drug. We can also say that the amount of homeopathic drugs given to the patients contains no drug at all.

References

Klaassen, C. D. (1980). Heavy metals and heavy metals antagonists. In A. G. Gilman, L. Goodman, & A. Gilman (Eds.), *Goodman and Gilman's pharmacological basis of therapeutics* (6th ed., pp. 1615–1637). New York, NY: Macmillan.

Krantz, J. C., & Carr, C. J. (1965). *The pharmacological principles of medical practice* (Indian 6th ed.). Baltimore, MD: Williams and Wilkins Company.

Modell, W., Schield, H., & Wilson, A. (1976). *Applied pharmacology* (American ed.). Toronto: W.B. Saunders Company.

Modi, N. J. (1975). *Textbook of medical jurisprudence and toxicology* (9th ed.). Bombay, India: N.M. Tripathi Publisher.

Srivastav, S. K. (2016). *Pharmacology for MBBS*. New Delhi, India: Avichal Publishing Company.

Ward, H. E., & Azzaro, A. J. (1997). Drugs used in mood disorders. In C. R. Craig, & R. E. Stitzel (Eds.), *Modern pharmacology with clinical application* (5th ed., pp. 385–396). Boston, MA: Little Brown and Company.

chapter three

Criticism of allopathy

Basic concept of homeopath – three

Hahnemann criticized allopathy. In allopathy, there were only a few treatments which were dangerous to human lives. In allopathy favorite remedies were bloodletting, emetics, and purgatives.

Argument

Hahnemann said in 1842 that allopathy was wrong. He criticized allopathy. Now here is a question: what was that allopathy which was criticized by Hahnemann? Was that modern medical science or some other methods of therapeutics? Followers of Hahnemann today criticize modern medical science on the basis of homeopathic principles. Are they correct or are they giving the wrong message to the public? These are very important questions that everybody should know.

Homeopathy word consists of homeo and patho, homeo = similar, patho = suffering. The symptoms produced by drugs are similar to symptoms of disease. That's why this system of therapeutics is known as homeopathy. Allopathy word consists of allo and pathos; here allo means different and pathos means suffering. Symptoms produced by drugs are different from those of disease. Therefore, this system of medicine was known as allopathy.

What was allopathy in the year 1800?

> In allopathy favorite remedies were bloodletting, emetics, and purgatives and these were used until the dominant symptoms of the disease were suppressed. Malaria and dysentery were treated by purging with calomel until collapse was produced. In a large proportion of cases, the suppression of the symptoms by collapse was followed shortly by death. (Modell et al., 1976, p. 9)

Medicinal leech therapy or hirudin therapy was a common form of therapy in various ailments. Sushruta Samhita, Ayurveda text, describes hirudin therapy (Singh & Rajoria, 2020). In the year 1827, bloodletting was

DOI: 10.1201/9781003228622-3

10   *Homeopathy*

performed by leeches in allopathy. Thirty-two million leeches were used in France. This system of allopathy was not based on adequate knowledge of physiology and pathology. This system was responsible for the death of many patients in place of cure. Bloodletting is also a part of Ayurveda. Leeches are used in Ayurveda for this purpose. Even today leeches are being used in Ayurveda hospitals in India for bloodletting. It has been said that many skin diseases are cured by this procedure and this application is a part of Ayurveda.

Hahnemann criticized allopathy because leeches were being used. Today leeches are being used in Ayurveda hospitals in India. Actually, Ayurveda was also a part of old allopathy that was criticized by Hahnemann. I am sorry to say that today people are accepting both Ayurveda and homeopathy without understanding that both are also opposite to each other.

Hahnemann rightly criticized allopathy. Hahnemann writes,

> Allopathy knows no treatment except to draw from diseases the injurious materials which are assumed to be their cause. The blood of the patient is made to flow mercilessly by bleedings, leeches, cuppings to diminish an assumed plethora (excess of blood) ... While the loss of blood ... destroys life. Allopathy taps off the life's blood and exerts itself either to clear away the imaginary disease matter or to conduct it elsewhere (by emetics, purgatives, diuretics, drawing plasters). This renders incurable if not fatal the majority of diseases. Patient's sufferings are thereby increased and by such and other painfull appliances the forces and nutritions juices indispensable to the curative process are abstracted from the organism. (Hahnemann, 1921/1993, pp. 15–17)

He has also written, "Allopathy has shortened the lives of ten times as many human beings as the most destructive wars and rendered many millions of patients more diseased and wretched than they were originally this allopathy" (Hahnemann, 1921/1993, p. 17).

Whatever Samuel Hahnemann said in 1840 about allopathy was right but what his followers are saying today is absolutely wrong. Today followers of homeopathy criticize modern medical science. They use allopathy words for it. This is wrong. Modern medical science is not related to old allopathy. The use of the term "allopathy" for modern medical science is wrong. But it is common practice to use the term allopathy for modern medical science. In fact, the principles of old allopathy are different from

Chapter three: Criticism of allopathy   *11*

modern medical science. The basis of old allopathy were not logical and not correct.

Medical science is based on logical controlled accurate experimentation, with full knowledge of pathogenesis of disease, pharmacokinetic and pharmacodynamic study of drugs. Hahnemann criticized allopathy in his work everywhere. This criticism is not related to modern medical science in any way.

Hahnemann writes, "Use of calomel, corrosive sublimate, mercurial ointment, nitrate of silver, iodine ointment, opium, valerian, cinchona bark and quinine, foxglove, prussic acid, sulfur and sulfuric acid, venesections, shedding streams of blood, leeches is dangerous to human body" (Hahnemann, 1921/1993, p. 162). These drugs and treatments were used by old allopathy. At present, in modern medical science, these treatments are not used systemically. Locally some compounds are used. Criticism of this treatment by Hahnemann is correct. But present medical science or present allopathy does not permit the use of these treatments. Only quinine and iodine are used systemically in malaria and hypothyroidism, respectively. Modern medical science uses iodine or quinine only after extensive study of 5–10 years on these compounds.

Hahnemann said about allopathy that this pathy is useless, cannot treat the disease, creates various problems in the body, and makes diseases incurable. He also said that innumerable abnormal conditions are produced by allopathy which cannot be treated (Hahnemann, 1921/1993, pp. 75–164). I am again and again saying that it was the criticism of the old allopathic mode of treatment. This criticism is right but not related to modern medical science which is also wrongly named allopathy today.

References

Hahnemann, S. (1993). *Organon of medicine* (6th ed.) (W. Boericke, Trans.). New Delhi, India: B. Jain Publishers. (Original work published in 1921).

Modell, W., Schield, H., & Wilson, A. (1976). *Applied pharmacology* (American ed.). Toronto, ON: W.B. Saunders Company.

Singh, S. K., & Rajoria, K. (2020). Medical leech therapy in Ayurveda and biomedicine – A review. *Journal of Ayurveda and Integrative Medicine, 11*(4), 554–564. https://doi.org/10.1016/j.jaim.2018.09.003.

chapter four

Knowledge regarding diseases

Basic concept of homeopathy – four

According to homeopathy, knowledge regarding etiology, pathology, and nature of disease is not important.

Argument

What Hahnemann emphasized in his first direction is,

> The physician's high and only mission is to restore the sick to health, to cure. His mission is not however to construct so called systems and hypothesis concerning the internal essential nature of the vital process and the mode in which diseases originate in the invisible interior of the organism, nor is it to attempt to give countless explanations regarding the phenomenon in diseases and their proximate cause. (Hahnemann, 1921/1993, p. 92)

According to homeopathy, knowledge and research regarding etiology, pathology, and nature of disease is not important. It is a waste of time and talent. Because of this homeopathy blocked the development of medical knowledge. In this way, questions against homeopathy cannot be raised on the basis of knowledge of developed medical science. It is ridiculous.

Etiology of disease is important to determine a method of treatment. Pathogenesis is important to know the accurate mechanism of symptomatology. Diagnosis of disease is also important to treat it accurately. Investigations are helpful in diagnosis. Discovery of new drugs also depends on detailed knowledge of diseases. Homeopathy opposes a detailed study of diseases. Without knowledge of etiology, prevention of disease cannot be possible. Today we know that the preventive aspect of disease is more important than the curative aspect. Many diseases such as AIDS and rabies have no cure. Only prevention of these diseases is possible and that can be done only on the basis of knowledge regarding

DOI: 10.1201/9781003228622-4

etiology and pathogenesis. All communicable diseases can be prevented in this manner. That modern medical science does, but homeopathy does not.

Reference

Hahnemann, S. (1993). *Organon of medicine* (6th ed.) (W. Boericke, Trans.). New Delhi, India: B. Jain Publishers. (Original work published in 1921).

chapter five

Nomenclature of diseases

Basic concept of homeopathy – five

Name and diagnosis of disease is not necessary. Nomenclature of diseases is not desired by this system. The knowledge of symptoms is sufficient.

Argument

Homeopathy says that name and diagnosis of disease is not necessary. Nomenclature of diseases is not required in this system. The knowledge of symptoms is sufficient in this therapy (Hahnemann, 1921/1996, p. 30). This indicates that diseases having common symptoms will be treated by the same drug. In homeopathy, etiology is not important for treatment purposes. Causative agents may be bacterial, fungal, hormonal, or carcinomatous, but treatment in homeopathy will remain the same. It is an illogical concept.

I am presenting one example. The diseases such as neurocysticercosis, tuberculoma of the brain, and neoplasm in the brain may have similar symptoms but their treatments are quite different.

Other important examples are headache, chest pain, dyspnea, and pain in abdomen. Each symptom has many causes that represent different diseases. Different diseases require different treatments. If all patients having similar symptoms are treated by the same drug, cure is never possible.

Reference

Hahnemann, S. (1996). *Organon of medicine* (6th ed.) (P. Devi, Trans.). New Delhi, India: B. Jain Publishers. (Original work published in 1921).

DOI: 10.1201/9781003228622-5

chapter six

Cures means removal of symptoms

Basic concept of homeopathy – six

Removal of symptoms means total cure. No symptom indicates no disease. Without symptoms the existence of disease in the body is not possible, homeopathy says.

Argument

The other basic concept of homeopathy is, "It is not conceivable, nor can it be proved by any experience in the world, that after removal of all the symptoms of the disease. . . there should or could remain anything else besides health" (Hahnemann, 1921/1993, p. 97). As mentioned above, if symptoms of a disease are removed, then disease is cured. Without symptoms disease cannot exist in the body. Nowadays, as we know from the study of the developed medical science, there are many diseases that have no symptoms at their early stage. During the early stage, pathogenesis starts. The healthy state of the body is changed, but there is no symptom. As disease advances, symptoms appear. Many diseases are episodic in nature. Between the episodes, the patient has no symptoms at all, although diseases persist in the body. Hypertension (a cardiovascular disease) may not produce any symptom even at an advanced stage because of that it has been called silent killer.

Similarly, a form of myocardial infarction called silent myocardial infarction is asymptomatic, although it may prove fatal. Carcinoma, diabetes, and degenerative neurological diseases do not have any symptoms during their early stages. Diseases such as asthma, epilepsy, angina, and peptic ulcer are episodic in nature with symptom-free periods between attacks.

Now it can be said that without symptoms, the existence of disease in the body is possible. It is against the basic concept of homeopathy.

Reference

Hahnemann, S. (1993). *Organon of medicine* (6th ed.) (W. Boericke, Trans.). New Delhi, India: B. Jain Publishers. (Original work published in 1921).

DOI: 10.1201/9781003228622-6

chapter seven

External factors for diseases

Basic concept of homeopathy – seven

Bacteria or other microbial agents, and any other external factors, are not responsible for development of disease. According to homeopathy, dirty food and dirty water cannot cause any disease.

Argument

One of the most important concepts of homeopathy is regarding causative factors of disease. According to homeopathy, bacteria are not causative factors in disease (Hahnemann, 1921/1996, p. 37).

Kent says, "The bacteria are results of disease.. . microscopical little fellows are not the disease cause, but that they come after, that they are scavengers accompanying the disease and that they are perfectly harmless in every respect. They are the outcome of the disease and present wherever the disease is" (Kent, 1993, p. 22).

Kent further states, "It is not from external things that man becomes sick, not from bacteria nor environment but from causes in himself. If the homeopath does not see this, he cannot have a true perception of disease. Disorder in the vital economy is the primary state of affairs and this disorder manifests itself by signs and symptoms" (Kent, 1993, p. 34).

> This concept of homeopathy is similar as expressed by YESHU MASIH in the Bible, New Testament, Mark. 7:14 – And turning to the people again, he said to them, Give ear to me all of you, and let my words be clear to you: 7:15 – There is nothing outside the man which, going into him, is able to make him unclean: but the things which come out of the man are those which make the man unclean. 7:16 and 7:17 – And when he had gone into the house away from all the people, his disciples put questions about the saying. 7:18 – And he said to them, Have you even a little wisdom? Do you not see that whatever goes into a man from outside is not able to make him unclean? 7:19 – Because it goes not into the heart

DOI: 10.1201/9781003228622-7

20 *Homeopathy*

> but into the stomach, and goes out with the waste? He said this, making all food clean. 7:20 – And he said, That which comes out of the man, that makes the man unclean. 7:21 – Because from inside, from the heart of men, come evil thoughts and unclean pleasures, 7:22 – The taking of goods and of life, broken faith between husband and wife, the desire of wealth, wrongdoing, deceit, sins of the flesh, an evil eye, angry words, pride, foolish acts: 7:23 – All these evil things come from inside, and make the man unclean. (Bible, Mark, 7.14–7.23)

Now it is clear that according to homeopathy, bacteria and other external agents like viruses, fungi, parasites, worms, and pollutants are not causative factors. Today it has been absolutely proven that bacteria, viruses, fungi, worms, and pollutants cause various diseases (Srivastava, 2016). In India, 75–85% diseases are caused by these agents. Typhoid, cholera, bacillary dysentery, pneumonia, respiratory tract infections, urinary tract infections, meningitis, tuberculosis, leprosy are common bacterial diseases, even a lay person knows that these are caused by bacteria. These diseases can only be treated by those drugs that kill responsible pathogens.

These are a few examples of bacteria responsible for disease. *Mycobacterium tuberculosis* causes tuberculosis, *Mycobacterium leprae* causes leprosy, Legionella causes legionnaires disease, *Calymmatobacterium granulomatis* causes granuloma inguinale, *Haemophilus ducreyi* causes chancroid, *Salmonella* bacteria causes typhoid fever, *Clostridium tetani* causes tetanus. Similarly other organisms such as spirochetes, fungus, virus, etc. also produce diseases. *Treponema pallidum* produces syphilis, *Treponema pertenue* produces yaws, *Leptospira* produces Weil's disease, *Chlamydia trachomatis* produces trachoma. Various viruses such as HIV produce AIDS disease, influenza virus produces influenza. In the absence of these organisms, respective diseases cannot be produced (Sande & Mandell, 1980, pp. 1085–1094).

Antibiotics are drugs used for killing these bacteria. Antibiotics kill bacteria because of that they are used in diseases caused by bacteria. Chloramphenicol, amoxicillin, and septran are used in typhoid because these drugs kill Salmonella bacteria. "Approximately 30% of all hospitalized patients receive one or more courses of therapy with antibiotics and millions of potentially fatal infections have been cured" (Sande & Mandell, 1980, p. 1081). "When an antimicrobial agent is indicated, the goal is to choose a drug that is selective for the infecting microorganism" (Sande & Mandell, 1980, p. 1085). "A large percentage of antibiotics administered in

Chapter seven: External factors for diseases 21

the United States are given to prevent infections rather than to treat established disease" (Sande & Mandell, 1980, p. 1100).

Now it is clear that antibiotics kill bacteria and cure diseases. Antibiotics also prevent development of disease in the body that's why they are also used for prophylaxis. It has also been proved by animal experiments that bacteria, viruses, fungi, and spirochaetes are responsible for various diseases. These are definite causative factors in disease production. Homeopathy says bacteria and virus-like organisms are not causative factors in disease. Now we can say this homeopathic concept is wrong. Pathology is the subject where pathogenesis is taught. Pathogenesis means how diseases are developed by bacteria, viruses, and other causative factors.

"Pathology is the study of disease by scientific methods. . . Disease may be defined as an abnormal variation in the structure or function of any part of the body" (Anderson, 1976, Introduction). Disease has causes. Causative factors in disease may be of a genetic nature or acquired. Acquired disease is due to effects of some external factors such as parasitic microorganisms, including bacteria, protozoa, lower fungi, and viruses. The disease-producing capacity of microorganisms depends on their capacity of invading and multiply within the host. Bacteria cause harmful effects mainly by toxins. It is also true that "Infective disease was the major cause of death throughout the world, and the elimination or reduction in the incidence of most of the important infections largely accounts for the greatly increased life span in technologically advanced communities" (Anderson, 1976, Introduction).

If bacteria are not responsible for diseases, then transmission of bacteria from one person to another person cannot produce similar disease but "Communicable disease is transmitted via direct transmission like direct contact, droplet infection, contact with soil, inoculation into skin and through placenta and via indirect transmission like vehicle borne, vector borne, airborne, fomite born and by unclean hands and fingers" (Park, 1997, p. 85). This proves that transmission of bacteria from one person to another produces similar disease.

Inoculation of bacteria in animals produces similar disease as produced in human beings and also confirms that bacteria cause disease. A person infected with HIV virus will develop AIDS and a person not infected with HIV virus will not develop AIDS, this also confirms the above statement. If it is confirmed in the lab that a particular bacteria is resistant to a drug, then this drug will not be effective in disease produced by that bacteria, which also gives the same conclusion.

Spread of communicable disease can also be checked by preventing transmission of etiological agents. Spread of cholera can be prevented by purifying contaminated food and water. Spread of malaria can be checked by preventing mosquito bite. If cholera, typhoid, and malaria originate from inside the body, then these diseases cannot be checked by preventing transmission of bacteria and malarial parasites.

Now a conclusion can be drawn that bacteria, virus, and parasites are definite causative factors in disease. Homeopathy says bacteria, virus, and any other external agents are not causative factors in disease. What does this indicate? This indicates that concepts of homeopathy are not correct.

References

Anderson, J. R. (1976). Introduction. In J. R. Anderson (Ed.), *Muir's textbook of pathology* (10th ed.). London, United Kingdom: ELBS & Edward Arnold.

Hahnemann, S. (1996). *Organon of medicine* (6th ed.) (P. Devi, Trans.). New Delhi, India: B. Jain Publishers. (Original work published in 1921).

Kent, J. T. (1993). *Lectures on homeopathic philosophy*. Delhi, India: B. Jain Publishers.

Park, K. (1997). *Park's textbook of preventive and social medicine* (15th ed.). Jabalpur, India: Banarsidas Bhanot Publisher.

Sande, M. A., & Mandell, G. L. (1980). Antimicrobial agents: General consideration. In A. G. Gilman, L. Goodman, & A. Gilman (Eds.), *Goodman and Gilman's pharmacological basis of therapeutics* (6th ed., pp. 1080–1105). New York, NY: Macmillan.

Srivastava, S. K. (2016). *Pharmacology for MBBS*. New Delhi, India: Avichal Publishing Company.

chapter eight

Rejection of pathological investigations

Basic concept of homeopathy – eight

Hahnemann rejected the examination of blood, urine, and other investigations for the diagnosis and treatment of disease.

Argument

Hahnemann says, "Totality of the symptoms is the only indication, the only guide to the selection of a remedy" (Hahnemann, 1921/1993, p. 21). On the basis of symptoms, drugs should be selected. There is no other alternative for drug selection. Hahnemann rejected the examination of blood, urine, and other investigation for the diagnosis and treatment of disease (Hahnemann, 1921/1996, p. 41).

Here, Hahnemann is absolutely wrong. There are various examples that are against this view. There are many causes of fever. "Bacterial, viral, malarial parasites, rickettsias, chlamydia are infections responsible for fever. Mechanical trauma, neoplasm, hematopoietic disorder, vascular accidents and acute metabolic disorder also cause fever" (Petersburg, 1983, p. 58).

Without complete investigation, it is not possible to diagnose fever, and without the accurate diagnosis, it is not possible to treat fever. The accurate diagnosis is only done on the basis of investigations. If somebody says that only on the basis of symptoms he can diagnose all diseases, this indicates that he does not know anything about the medical science.

Similar to fever, there are many diseases having common symptoms that cannot be treated without the accurate diagnosis and such diagnosis solely depends on various investigations.

Hahnemann writes,

> Physicians can discover diseases consists … solely of the totality of the symptoms by means of which the disease demands the medicine requisite for its relief, whilst on the other hand every internal cause attributed to it, every occult quality or imaginary

DOI: 10.1201/9781003228622-8

24   *Homeopathy*

material morbific principle is nothing but an idle
dream. (Hahnemann, 1921/1993, pp. 156–157)

According to homeopathy, there is no need to diagnose any internal
cause of disease and any external bacteria or virus. The examination of
symptoms is sufficient. For example, if a patient is suffering from abdominal pain, then there is no need for an ultrasound or X-ray.

Investigations of particular disease are not required in homeopathy.
Abdominal pain may be due to pathology in the liver, pancreas, stomach,
duodenum, uterus, ovary, cardiac, or muscular organs. In homeopathy, it
is not required to know which organ is responsible for pain, and it is also
undesirable to know which organ has pathology. Irrespective of organ
pathology and the cause in homeopathy, the treatment of abdominal pain
remains constant. And in this therapy, treatment would be done by the
drug that will cause abdominal pain in the healthy body.

In tropical countries such as India, conditions are quite different. In
tropical countries, the maximum number of diseases is due to microorganisms. In viral and bacterial diseases, immunity plays an important
role in recovery. Viral diseases usually resolve spontaneously. This is also
true for many bacterial diseases. Many sexually transmitted diseases are
also cured spontaneously. When diseases are going to be cured spontaneously, then neither diagnosis nor treatment is important. In these diseases,
like homeopathy many other systems get an unnecessary reputation as
curative methods without having any useful therapeutic action. Because
of this, Hahnemann got an unnecessary reputation and he formulated the
wrong concept that the examination of symptoms is sufficient and investigations are not required.

References

Hahnemann, S. (1993). *Organon of medicine* (6th ed.) (W. Boericke, Trans.).
New Delhi, India: B. Jain Publishers. (Original work published in 1921).
Hahnemann, S. (1996). *Organon of medicine* (6th ed.) (P. Devi, Trans.). New Delhi,
India: B. Jain Publishers. (Original work published in 1921).
Petersburg, R. G. (1983). Chills and fever. In R. G. Petersdorf, R. D. Adams, E.
Braunwald, K. J. Isselbacher, J. B. Martin, & J. D. Wilson (Eds.), *Harrison's
principle of internal medicine* (10th ed., pp. 57–65). New Delhi, India:
McGraw Hill.

chapter nine

Mechanism of cure

Basic concept of homeopathy – nine

Medicines can show nothing curative besides their tendency to produce morbid symptoms in healthy persons and to remove them in diseased persons.

Argument

Homeopathy says, "It is very evident that medicine could never cure diseases if they did not possess the power of altering man's state of health. Their curative power must be owing solely to this power they possess of altering man's state of health" (Hahnemann, 1921/1993, p. 106). Homeopathy also says that "Medicines can show nothing curative besides their tendency to produce morbid symptoms in healthy persons and to remove them in diseased persons" (Hahnemann, 1921/1993, p. 107).

This indicates that, according to homeopathy, if a drug is not able to produce side effects in a healthy person, it will not be able to cure disease. But Ayurveda says that Ayurvedic drugs do not have any side effects, and these drugs have only therapeutic effects. This is a contradiction between Ayurvedic and homeopathic drugs. But people accept Ayurveda and homeopathy both without any logical thinking.

According to homeopathy, there are two different systems of treatment. One is homeopathy where symptoms produced by drugs in a healthy body are similar to symptoms of disease. In another system, symptoms produced by drugs in a healthy body are neither similar or opposite but quite heterogeneous to symptoms of disease. This other system is known as the allopathic method of therapy.

Allopathic methods of treatment include Ayurveda and Unani systems (Hahnemann, 1921/1996, p. 18). Here again homeopathy and Ayurveda have opposite concepts, but people accept and favor both Ayurveda and homeopathy without knowing the basics.

Homeopathy also says, "Nothing can be observed that can constitute medicine or remedies except that power of causing distinct alteration on the state of health of the human body" (Hahnemann, 1921/1993, p. 107). In 1833 when Hahnemann wrote *Organon of Medicine*, there was nothing except development of morbid symptoms in healthy body by a drug to

DOI: 10.1201/9781003228622-9

25

test its therapeutic capability because in that time there were no biochemical tests, no histopathological study, no culture and sensitivity study, no biopsy, no X-rays, no ultrasound, and no MRI. In the absence of knowledge, Hahnemann made hypothetical and philosophical concepts that were not based on scientific observations. Therapeutic potency of a drug cannot be evaluated by morbid alteration in a healthy body.

Hahnemann writes,

> Each individual case of disease is most surely, radically, rapidly and permanently annihilated and removed only by a medicine capable of producing in the human system in the most similar and complete manner the totality of its symptoms, which at the same time are stronger than the disease. (Hahnemann, 1921/1993, p. 112)

Hahnemann writes, "No other mode of employing medicines in diseases that promises to be of service besides the homeopathic ... a medicine which among all medicines has the power and the tendency to produce an artificial morbid state most similar to that of the case of disease" (Hahnemann, 1921/1993, p. 109).

Today we have various examples of drugs that do not prove the homeopathic concept. Antipsychotic drugs like chlorpromazine and thioridazine are useful in schizophrenia, but when these drugs are given to healthy individuals they never produce symptoms of schizophrenia. Similarly, antidepressant drugs like imipramine and amitriptyline used in depression never produce depression in healthy persons. Antacids are used in hyperacidity, and these drugs never produce hyperacidity in healthy individuals. Various antibiotics like ampicillin and erythromycins are used in respiratory tract infections, but they never develop symptoms of respiratory infections in healthy people. Similarly, there are various examples that prove that homeopathic concepts given above are wrong. Antileprosy drugs cure leprosy, but never produce leprosy in healthy persons. Antitubercular drugs cure tuberculosis but never produce the symptoms of tuberculosis when given to a healthy person. Antihypertensive drugs never produce hypertensive states when given to a healthy body. Drugs used in pain like brufen never produce pain in healthy humans.

Similarly, the combination of trimethoprim and sulfamethoxazole is useful in typhoid, but this combination never produces symptoms of typhoid when given to healthy individuals. Another example is ciprofloxacin that is used in many diseases related to the urinary tract, prostate, respiratory tract, bone, and gastrointestinal tract, but it never produces symptoms of these diseases (Satoskar et al., 2011).

Chapter nine: Mechanism of cure 27

Hahnemann further writes, medicine should be capable of producing an artificial disease in the human body as similar as possible to the disease to be cured with somewhat increased power (Hahnemann, 1921/1996, p. 52).

As indicated in the above examples that drugs useful in a particular disease neither produce symptoms of that disease in healthy individuals nor produce artificial disease, similar to the disease to be cured. In this way, we can say that these above statements of Hahnemann are not correct.

References

Hahnemann, S. (1993). *Organon of medicine* (6th ed.) (W. Boericke, Trans.). New Delhi, India: B. Jain Publishers. (Original work published in 1921).

Hahnemann, S. (1996). *Organon of medicine* (6th ed.) (P. Devi, Trans.). New Delhi, India: B. Jain Publishers. (Original work published in 1921).

Satoskar, R. S., Rege, N. N., & Bhandarkar, S. D. (2011). *Pharmacology and pharmacotherapeutics* (22nd ed.). Mumbai, India: Popular Prakashan.

chapter ten

Interaction of diseases

Basic concept of homeopathy – ten

Two dissimilar diseases cannot remove, cannot cure one another. Stronger disease only suspends dissimilar weaker disease.

Argument

Hahnemann writes, "If new dissimilar disease is stronger than the disease under which the patient originally labored being the weaker will be kept back and suspended by the accession of the stronger one, until the later shall have run its course or been cured and then the old one reappears uncured" (Hahnemann, 1921/1993, p. 118). I am continuously emphasizing that in medical science we can't draw any conclusion by using few examples. It could be by chance. For example, "Hahnemann quoted, two children affected with a kind of epilepsy remained free from epileptic attacks after infection with ringworm but as soon as eruption on head was gone the epilepsy returned just as before" (Hahnemann, 1921/1993, p. 118). Here Hahnemann made the wrong conclusion of suspension of epilepsy by ringworm. The fact is different. Actually in epilepsy, attack occurs intermittently with the gap of days, weeks, or months. It is the natural course of the disease. During the middle silent stage of epilepsy, if ringworm appears and subsides, then how the relation between epilepsy and ringworm can be established. To establish such a relationship is useless.

Hahnemann made some observations of infectious diseases. He found that sometimes one disease suspended another disease and sometimes one disease cured another disease. He did not know the mechanism of immunity and antigen antibody reaction, which plays the main part in suspending and curing one disease by another. The important points of this process are as follows:

1. Following immunization (or by a disease), there may occur a disease totally unconnected with the immunizing agent (or disease-producing agent). Actually the individual is harboring the infectious agent and administration of vaccine or exposure to disease shortens the incubation period and produces the disease in such cases.

DOI: 10.1201/9781003228622-10

30   *Homeopathy*

2. If many antigens are administered in an animal at the same time, the antibody response to each may be less than that if the antigens are introduced individually.

3. "Recovery is of course the rule in the vast majority of viral infections" (Pinkerton, 1971, p. 376).

4. Cox virus and smallpox virus have common antigens and give immunity to each other.

5. One or few observations do not give any clue.

6. First we should know the normal course of the disease, then only we can study the influence of other factors on the disease process.

7. "Many infections (Viral) are entirely symptomless and immunity to reinfection is acquired without serious disturbance at the time of primary infection although latent infection with virus may continue for months or occasionally even for years" (Anderson, 1976, p. 161).

8. "Persistent virus infections are known to occur in men. . . Slow virus infections may be defined as virus disease having a long incubation period, in some instance years ... In a few virus diseases reinfection or repeated infections are common. This may be due to the existence of numerous serologically distinct strains of virus" (Anderson, 1976, p. 162).

9. "Virus infections occur with disease or asymptomatics. The severity of disease may also be age related. In adults chicken pox and mumps are often severe with complications which are rare during childhood" (Lerner, 1983, p. 1095).

10. "If common exposure of viral infection to several persons occurs, illness may be simultaneous irrespective of the length of the incubation period" (Lerner, 1983, p. 1096).

11. Diagnosis of viral disease is only done by isolation or recognition of virus and by the help of specific serological tests.

12. "In the acute phase of virus infections a protein interferon can be detected in blood and tissue. Interferon is released from cells in response to virus infections and when taken up by other cells make them refractory to virus infection. It is not virus specific in its antiviral effect but inhibits virtually all viruses. It begins to appear in the bloodstream only when the acute infection is subsiding" (Anderson, 1976, p. 161).

Using the above given information we can understand the causes of the varied incubation period, duration, intensity, and prognosis of a disease when a patient also suffers with another disease. In favor of his opinion Hahnemann writes, "during an epidemic, in which smallpox and

Chapter ten: Interaction of diseases 31

measles were prevalent at the same time, these diseases avoided or suspended one another" (Hahnemann, 1921/1996, p. 124). Actually, both are viral infections and interferon produced by acute viral infection prevented or suspended another viral infection.

Simultaneous occurrences of small pox and measles also occur at the same time as written by Hahnemann (Hahnemann, 1921/1996, pp. 166–167). In this case, interferon is not in sufficient amounts, which could have suspended a second infection. In another case, "Measles suspended the cowpox" (Hahnemann, 1921/1993, p. 120). In another example, "Even after measles had broken out the cowpox inoculation took effect but did not run its course until the measles had disappeared" (Hahnemann, 1921/1993, p. 120). In other examples, "Mumps immediately disappeared when the cowpox inoculation had taken effect and had nearly attained its height, it was not until the complete termination of the cowpox ... mumps reappeared and ran its regular course of seven days" (Hahnemann, 1921/1993, p. 120).

Hahnemann also writes, "Smallpox causes swelling of testicles and in one observation a large hard swelling of the left testicle consequent on a bruise is cured by smallpox" (Hahnemann, 1921/1993, p. 129). It is a normal observation that after trauma swelling anywhere in the body is resolved automatically. Similarly, swelling in testicle after trauma cured automatically. This cure is not related to smallpox. The relation between swelling induced by trauma and small pox infection is incorrect. Other examples mentioned by Hahnemann in favor of his view are being analyzed in the last part of this book.

One viral infection may suspend or prevent a second subsequent infection due to common antigenic structure or release of interferon. Similarity and dissimilarity of symptomatology in these two diseases are not important. Only those infective organisms that produce interferon may prevent another viral infection because interferon has antiviral action. Many infective and noninfective diseases having dissimilar symptomatology coexist together in the body. Again Hahnemann made the wrong generalization of a few observations.

References

Anderson, J. R. (1976). Type of infection. In J. R. Anderson (Ed.), *Muir's textbook of pathology* (10th ed., pp. 160–190). London, United Kingdom: ELBS & Edward Arnold.

Hahnemann, S. (1993). *Organon of medicine* (6th ed.) (W. Boericke, Trans.). New Delhi, India: B. Jain Publishers. (Original work published in 1921).

Hahnemann, S. (1996). *Organon of medicine* (6th ed.) (P. Devi, Trans.). New Delhi, India: B. Jain Publishers. (Original work published in 1921).

Lerner, A. M. (1983). An overview of viral infection. In R. G. Petersdorf, R. D. Adams, E. Braunwald, K. J. Isselbacher, J. B. Martin, & J. D. Wilson (Eds.), *Harrison's principle of internal medicine* (10th ed., pp. 1091–1098). New Delhi, India: McGraw Hill.

Pinkerton, H. (1971). Rickettsial, chlamydia and viral diseases. In W. A. D. Anderson (Ed.), *Pathology* (6th ed., pp. 365–408). St Louis, MO: C. V. Mosby Company.

chapter eleven

Causes of chronic diseases

Basic concept of homeopathy – eleven

There are only three causes of all chronic diseases: syphilis, sycosis, and psora.

Argument

Hahnemann says that there are three fundamental causes of all chronic diseases: (a) syphilis, (b) sycosis, and (c) psora. Hahnemann further says that even after the treatment of skin eruption of syphilis and sycosis, seeds of these diseases remain inside the body and continuously create problems. Syphilis reveals its specific internal dyscrasia by venereal chancre and sycosis by cauliflower-like growth and sometimes skin eruption with itching. Third, psora is a more dangerous seed than syphilis and sycosis (Hahnemann, 1921/2017, p. 117).

> The psora, the psora is the only real fundamental cause and producer of all other numerous, I may say innumerable, forms of disease, which under the names of nervous debility, hysteria, hypochondriasis, mania, melancholia, imbecility, madness, epilepsy, convulsion of all sorts, softening of bone, scoliosis and kyphosis, caries, cancer, fungus haematodes,neoplasm, gout, haemorrhoids, jaundice cyanosis, dropsy, amenorrhoea, haemorrhage from the stomach, nose, lungs, bladder and womb, of asthma and ulceration of lungs, of impotence and barrenness, of megrim, deafness, cataract, amaurosis, urinary calculus, paralysis, defects of the senses, pains of thousands of kinds etc. are due to psora. (Hahnemann, 1921/2017, p. 117)

At the time of Hahnemann around 1800, medical science was not developed. Causative agent, pathogenesis, method of spread, and prognosis were not known. That's why Hahnemann concluded wrongly that all chronic diseases are caused by only one agent, psora. Actually, all diseases

DOI: 10.1201/9781003228622-11

mentioned by Hahnemann have different causes. All students of biology and medical science know this fact. It is not correct to accept one cause of all diseases. Even today in homeopathic colleges, it is being taught.

Reference

Hahnemann, S. (2017). *Organon of medicine* (6th ed.) (W. Boericke, Trans.). New Delhi, India: B. Jain Publishers. (Original work published in 1921).

chapter twelve

Change the drug treatment

Basic concept of homeopathy – twelve

If symptoms of disease are changed, then drugs should be changed.

Argument

Homeopathic treatment is based on the symptoms of disease. If symptoms are not seen, then homeopathy will not suggest any treatment. According to this pathy, if symptoms are not present, then there is no treatment because the drug is chosen only on the basis of similar symptoms produced in a healthy person when the drug is given.

In hypertension and the early stages of cancer, open angle glaucoma, diabetes, there are no symptoms. Homeopathy will not suggest any treatment in these conditions. When diseases advance and conditions of patients deteriorate, then only homeopathy provides treatment on the basis of presenting symptoms. Those Diseases in which symptoms are not presented, homeopathy does not suggest any treatment.

Hahnemann writes, during the treatment, the symptoms of disease should be studied. If the symptoms are changed or new symptoms appear, then drugs should be changed (Hahnemann, 1921/2017, pp. 132–134).

Homeopathy emphasizes only on symptoms. There are various diseases in which symptoms in early stages are different than those in late stages. Examples of such diseases are syphilis, tuberculosis, cancer, diabetes, and glaucoma. According to homeopathy, treatments at early stages will be different from the treatment at late stages.

Treatments of syphilis, diabetes, tuberculosis, and cancer are very specific irrespective of stage of disease. The same treatment is given whether disease is at early stage or at advanced stage. So, the importance given to only symptoms by homeopathy is absolutely wrong.

Reference

Hahnemann, S. (2017). *Organon of medicine* (6th ed.) (W. Boericke, Trans.). New Delhi, India: B. Jain Publishers. (Original work published in 1921).

DOI: 10.1201/9781003228622-12

chapter thirteen

Only homeopathy is best

Basic concept of homeopathy – thirteen

Hahnemann said that only homeopathy can cure diseases. Those who believe that there are other therapeutic methods also do not understand homeopathy.

Argument

Hahnemann said,

> It is impossible that there can be another true, best method of curing dynamic disease, besides homeopathy, just as it is impossible to draw more than one straight line between two given points. He who imagines that there are other modes of curing diseases besides it, could not have appreciated homeopathy fundamentally, nor practiced it with sufficient care, nor could he ever have seen or read cases of properly performed homeopathic cures … My true, conscientious followers, the pure homeopathists, with their successful, almost never failing treatment, might teach these persons better. (Hahnemann, 1921/2017, pp. 135–136)

Homeopathy says that all other therapeutic methods are wrong, and the followers of homeopathy should not use any other therapeutic methods.

Then the government should discard modern medical science and Ayurveda from society if it is really a supporter of homeopathy. Followers of homeopathy should never use modern medical science in their lifetime, if they are really the followers of homeopathy.

Reference

Hahnemann, S. (2017). *Organon of medicine* (6th ed.) (W. Boericke, Trans.). New Delhi, India: B. Jain Publishers. (Original work published in 1921).

DOI: 10.1201/9781003228622-13

chapter fourteen

Curative power of medicine

Basic concept of homeopathy – fourteen

All the curative power of medicines lies in the power they possess of changing the state of man's health and is revealed by observation of the latter. Hahnemann recommended a drug of 30th potency for such studies.

Argument

Hahnemann writes,

> Business of a true physician relates to acquiring a knowledge of the instruments intended for the cure of natural diseases, investigating the pathogenic power of the medicines, in order, when called on to cure … The whole pathogenic effect of the several medicines must be known, that is to say all the morbid symptoms and alteration in the health that each of them is especially capable of developing in the healthy individual must first have been observed as far as possible before we can hope to be able to find among them and to select suitable homeopathic remedies for most of the natural diseases. (Hahnemann, 1921/2017, pp. 133–134)

He also said,

> Peculiar powers of medicines available for cure of disease are to be learned neither by any ingenious a priori speculations nor by the smell, taste, appearance of the drugs nor by their chemical analysis, nor yet by the employment of several of them at one time in a mixture (prescription) in diseases. (Hahnemann, 1921/1993, p. 191)

Hahnemann had a firm opinion that the curative power of drugs cannot be determined by studying them in patients. According to him, studying (chemical or physical) drugs is also useless.

DOI: 10.1201/9781003228622-14

40   *Homeopathy*

If these concepts of determination of curative power of drugs are correct, then all experimental studies should be stopped. Research and development of new drugs would be useless. According to homeopathy, drug development is very easy. Administer a compound in a healthy individual and observe symptoms. That is sufficient. Hahnemann prescribed a method of studying the curative power of drugs in healthy humans.

> Medicinal substances ... are taken for the same object in high dilutions potentized by proper trituration and succussion by which simple operations the powers which in their crude state lay hidden and as it were dormant, are developed and roused into activity to an incredible extent ... The plan we adopted is to give to the experimenter on an empty stomach, daily from four to six very small globules of the thirtieth potency of such a substance moistened with a little water or dissolved in more or less water and thoroughly mixed and let him continue this for several days. (Hahnemann, 1921/2017, p. 145)

Hahnemann prescribed a drug in the 30th potency. Thirtieth potency means 1 in 10^{60} dilution. With this dilution, what I am saying there will not be any effect on the human body because this concentration does not contain a single molecule of a drug. By this dilution, nothing can be observed. But what was observed by Hahnemann? He observed many pathological effects of drugs in a healthy body. If we observe and analyze minutely what was observed by Hahnemann, it is not accurate. His observations were false.

He writes,

> For all persons are not affected by a medicine in an equally great degree; on the contrary there is a vast variety in this respect, so that sometimes an apparently weak individual may be scarcely at all affected by moderate dose of a medicine known to be of a powerful character whilst he is strongly enough acted on by others of a much weaker kind and, on the other hand, there are very robust persons who experience very considerable morbid symptoms from an apparently mild medicine and only slight symptom from stronger drugs. (Hahnemann, 1921/1993, p. 202)

Hahnemann said during this study, sometimes severe morbid symptoms are produced and sometimes by similar drug only mild symptoms

Chapter fourteen: Curative power of medicine 41

are developed. He also said, "Among these symptoms, they occur in the case of some medicines, not a few which are partially or under certain conditions directly opposite to other symptoms that have previously or subsequently appeared" (Hahnemann, 1921/1993, p. 194).

"Subsequent dose often removes curatively some one or other of the symptoms caused by the previous dose or develops in its stead an opposite state" (Hahnemann, 1921/1993, p. 203).

He also writes,

> All the symptoms peculiar to a medicine do not appear in one person, nor all at once, nor in the same experiment but some occur in one person chiefly at one time, others again during a second or third trial, in another person some other symptoms appear but in such a manner than probably some of the phenomena are observed in the fourth, eight, or tenth person which had already appeared in the second, sixth or ninth person and so forth; moreover they may not recur at the same hour. (Hahnemann, 1921/1993, p. 205)

He also said that it is very rare to develop all symptoms of a drug in a medium who is a healthy person (Hahnemann, 1921/1996, p. 139).

Above description indicates that there is no consistency in the development of symptoms by experimental drugs. There is a vast variety in this respect. The same dose produces sometimes strong symptoms and sometimes opposite symptoms. All symptoms of a drug are not produced in a single person. Different symptoms are produced in different persons at different times by different doses. This indicates there is no uniformity and consistency in symptoms, which should be, if there is definite correlation between drug and symptoms. I am saying again and again that drugs of such dilution cannot produce symptoms. Is it possible that symptoms can be produced without giving any drug just by suggestion? Yes. The study proved that symptoms can be produced without giving any drug.

> Studies have shown that about 80% of healthy people not taking any drug admit to questioning symptoms (often several) such as commonly experienced as lesser adverse reactions to drugs ... Therefore to avoid misinterpretation these symptoms are intensified (or diminished) by administration of a placebo ... Thus many symptoms may be wrongly attributed to drugs. (Laurence & Bennett, 1992, pp. 120–121)

A dose response curve should be determined to know the definite qualitative action of a drug in different subjects. For the definite amount of action, minimum dose should be known. Certainty and persistence in different subjects prove the relation between drug and response.

> Minimum pharmacological effect will occur in all subjects when a certain amount of drug has been administered ... augmented reactions will occur in every one if enough of the drug is given because they are due to excess of normal predictable dose related pharmacodynamic effects. (Laurence & Bennett, 1992, pp. 120–121)

With dilution of the 30th potency, uniform and persistent symptoms were not found by Hahnemann and studies also show that without prescribing drugs, symptoms can be produced. We also know that drugs of this dilution contain no drug molecules. For a pharmacological action, a minimum amount of drug is necessary. Now we can say that the symptoms observed by Hahnemann with drugs of 30th potency were not related to drugs. It also means that the concept of homeopathy regarding proving of drug by giving 30th potency is wrong. Even if drug has been proved by giving concentrated form, this does not mean that this drug will be effective in disease having similar symptomatology. And it is also true when drug is given in homeopathic doses, it has no curative effect.

Kent also writes,

> Each prover takes a single dose of the medicine and waits to see if the single dose takes effect ... If we were attempting to prove a remedy like silicate of alumina. The master prover would advise the class not to interfere with the medicine for at least thirty days because its prodrome may be thirty days. (Kent, 1993, p. 186)

Here Kent advised for a thirty-day observation for proving a drug.

Pharmacokinetic knowledge is also important to get accurate conclusions. Orally giving drug in a single dose only cannot remain in the gastrointestinal lumen for more than 48 hours. Either it will absorb from the gastrointestinal or it will pass out with stool. After absorption, the drug reaches the blood and then there will be an onset of action. After that metabolism and excretion start. The peak effect on the body diminishes gradually. Drugs may remain in the body up to months but the maximum peak effect will occur within a week, it cannot be delayed. Pharmacokinetic

Chapter fourteen: Curative power of medicine   43

study means a study regarding drug absorption, drug metabolism, and excretion. Each drug has a different pharmacokinetic character and this knowledge is needed to establish relation between drug and symptomatology it produces. If an orally administered drug in a single dose only produces action after seven days of its administration, this indicates that such action has no relation with the orally administered drug. These symptoms must be due to some other cause or just psychological. Kent, Hahnemann, and other homeopaths made this mistake. Hahnemann and Kent never recommended the study of homeopathy drugs in patients. They recommended study of symptoms produced by drugs in a healthy body only. Now it is clear that the method used by Hahnemann and Kent for proving the drug is absolutely wrong.

References

Hahnemann, S. (1993). *Organon of medicine* (6th ed.) (W. Boericke, Trans.). New Delhi, India: B. Jain Publishers. (Original work published in 1921).

Hahnemann, S. (1996). *Organon of medicine* (6th ed.) (P. Devi, Trans). New Delhi, India: B. Jain Publishers. (Original work published in 1921).

Hahnemann, S. (2017). *Organon of medicine* (6th ed.) (W. Boericke, Trans.). New Delhi, India: B. Jain Publishers. (Original work published in 1921).

Kent, J. T. (1993). *Lectures on homeopathic philosophy.* Delhi, India: B. Jain Publishers.

Laurence, D. R., & Bennett, P. N. (1992). *Clinical pharmacology* (7th ed.). Harlow, United Kingdom: Churchill Livingstone.

chapter fifteen

Displacement of pathological symptoms

Basic concept of homeopathy – fifteen

If artificial diseases produced by drugs are more powerful than the diseases to be treated, then only it can displace pathological symptoms of disease.

Argument

Hahnemann defined primary and secondary action.

> Every agent that acts upon the vitality, every medicine deranges more or less the vital force and causes a certain alteration in the health of the individual for a longer or shorter period. This is termed primary action ... To its action our vital force endeavors to oppose its own energy. This resistant action is indeed an automatic action of our life preserving power, which goes by the name of secondary action or counteraction. (Hahnemann, 1921/2017, p. 102)

Hahnemann has also written some examples of primary and secondary action.

> A hand bathed in hot water is at first much warmer than the other hand that has not been so treated (Primary action); but when it is withdrawn from the hot water and again thoroughly dried it becomes in a short time cold and at length much colder than the other (secondary action). A person heated by violent exercise (primary action) is afterwards affected with chilliness and shivering (Secondary action). To one who was yesterday heated by drinking much wine (primary action), today every breath of air feels too cold (counter action of the organism,

DOI: 10.1201/9781003228622-15

45

46   *Homeopathy*

> secondary action). An arm that has been kept long
> in very cold water is at first much paler and colder
> (Primary action) than the other, but removed from
> the cold water and dried, it subsequently becomes
> warmer, hot red. (Hahnemann, 1921/1993, p. 150)

This secondary action or counteraction is the reaction of the body against the primary action to sustain homeostasis. Body has the capacity to maintain normal equilibrium in the body.

Hahnemann writes,

> when a person falls ill, it is only this spiritual, self
> acting (automatic) vital force, everywhere present
> in his organism, that is primarily deranged by the
> dynamic influence up on it of a morbific agent inim-
> ical to life; it is only the vital principle deranged to
> such an abnormal state, that can furnish the organ-
> ism with its disagreeable sensations and incline
> it to the irregular process which we call disease.
> (Hahnemann, 1921/2017, pp. 58–59)

Vital force tries to control the diseases. If the causes of diseases are strong, then only vital force does not suppress them and the diseases are developed (Hahnemann, 1921/1996, p. 50). He also writes,

> It is only the slighter and acute diseases that
> tend. When the natural period of their course has
> expired, to terminate quietly in resolution as it is
> called with or without the employment of not very
> aggressive allopathic remedies, the vital force hav-
> ing regained its power, then gradually substitutes
> the normal condition for the derangement of the
> health that has now ceased to exist. But in severe
> acute and chronic diseases which constitute by for
> the greater portion of the all human ailments crude
> nature and the old school are equally powerless, in
> these neither the vital force with its self aiding fac-
> ulty, nor allopathy in imitation of it. (Hahnemann,
> 1921/1993, p. 52)

Hahnemann was correct about the concept that vital power and natural capacity of the body help in fighting the disturbance of the body and try to maintain normal equilibrium.

Chapter fifteen: Displacement of pathological symptoms 47

> Normal cell function depends on the constancy of this fluid, it is not surprising that in multicellular animals an immense number of regulatory mechanisms have evolved to maintain it. To describe the various physiological arrangements which serve to restore the normal state, once it has been disturbed. W.B. Cannon coined the term homeostasis … Many of these regulatory mechanisms operate on the principle of negative feedback, deviations from a given normal set point are detected by a sensor, and signals from the sensor trigger compensatory changes that continue until the set point is again reached. (Ganong, 2003, p. 48)

> As long as normal conditions are maintained in this internal environment, the cells of the body continue to live and function property … Extreme dysfunction leads to death whereas moderate dysfunction leads to sickness. (Vaz, 2016, pp. 7–8)

Hahnemann gives emphasis to the curative power of vital force. Hahnemann stated that slighter and acute diseases are resolved spontaneously. If disturbing agents are of shorter duration, then they can be controlled easily by compensatory mechanisms of the body. When homeostasis fails, disease starts. Symptomatology of disease develops only when homeostasis fails.

Hahnemann said, "A weaker dynamic affection is permanently extinguished in the living organism by a stronger one, if the latter (whilst differing in kind) is very similar to the former in its manifestations" (Hahnemann, 1921/1993, p. 111).

> The curative power of medicines therefore depends on their symptoms similar to the disease but superior to it in strength, So that each individual case of disease is most surely radically, rapidly and permanently annihilated and removed only by a medicine capable of producing (in the human system) in the most similar and complete manner the totality of its symptoms which at the same time are stronger than the disease. (Hahnemann, 1921/1993, p. 112)

Hahnemann stated that natural disease can be cured by homeopathic drugs, which produce similar symptoms as produced by disease. But Hahnemann was wrong. Disease already has disturbed homeostasis.

48   *Homeopathy*

Similar symptoms, if produced by drug, will further disturb the homeo-stasis. Then the vital force of the body cannot compensate. Homeopathic drugs by creating similar symptomatology will deteriorate the vital capac-ity of the body further. Disease cannot be cured by this method. Actually, homeopathic drugs used in such dilutions can never produce symptoms in a healthy body. If homeopathic drugs produce symptoms in a healthy body, then disease will definitely be aggravated. For example, "leptazol is a compound that is commonly used to produce convulsion. It is usually injected subcutaneously as a 1 percent solution in the dose of 100 mg/kg body weight" (Satoskar & Bhandarkar, 1988, p. 102). It will be impossible to cure an epileptic patient by giving leptazol in such doses that produces convulsion. There will be death in place of cure, if leptazol is given dur-ing convulsion. Similarly, we can say by this mechanism diseases can-not be cured, they can aggravate only. According to Hahnemann, leptazol will be the best drug in epilepsy when given in the 30th potency, but things are not like this. Invention of drugs is not so simple. Hahnemann was wrong. He also did not explain how pathological symptoms can cure the disease of similar symptoms. He knew his limitations, that's why he writes, "It matters little what may be the scientific explanation of how it takes place and I do not attach much importance to the attempts made to explain it" (Hahnemann, 1921/1993, p. 112). His arguments in this favor are ridiculous.

> The stronger disease, namely, annihilates the weaker and that for simple reason, because the stronger morbific power when it invades the sys-tem by reason of its similarity of action involves precisely the same parts of the organism that were previously affected by the weaker morbid imita-tion, which consequently can no longer act on these parts, but is extinguished just as the image of lamp's flame is rapidly overpowered and effaced from our retina by the stronger sunbeam impinging on the eye. (Hahnemann, 1921/1993, p. 128)

Such philosophical arguments have no place in science.

Regarding this matter Hahnemann was confused, that's why he gave contradictory statements. At one place, he writes that artificial disease produced by homeopathic drugs is more powerful than natural dis-ease (Hahnemann, 1921/1996, p. 52). "According to nature, disease can be removed solely by one that is similar in symptoms and is somewhat stronger" (Hahnemann, 1921/1993, p. 133). In another place, Hahnemann writes, in homeopathic cure after the removal of natural disease, "a certain

Chapter fifteen: Displacement of pathological symptoms 49

amount of medicinal disease remain in the organism but on account of the extra minuteness of the dose, it is so transient, so slight and disappears so rapidly of its own accord that the vital force has no need to employ against this small artificial derangement of its health" (Hahnemann, 1921/1993, p. 153).

Hahnemann writes at one point that artificial symptoms produced by homeopathic drugs are stronger and powerful than natural disease, while at another place he writes that during homeopathic treatment, extraordinary minuteness of the dose of homeopathic drug produces transient and slight symptoms that disappear spontaneously. Hahnemann did not explain the cause of this contradiction. He mentioned only that after the removal of disease symptoms, symptoms produced by homeopathic drugs become very mild (Hahnemann, 1921/1996, pp. 89–90). How does it take place? What is the logic behind this comment, nothing has been said?

At one point Hahnemann writes, "Excessively minute dose requisite for homeopathic use is much too weak to produce the other symptoms of the medicine that are not homeopathic to case in those parts of the body that are free from disease" (Hahnemann, 1921/1993, p. 219). In this paragraph, Hahnemann said homeopathic drugs have no effect on healthy organs. It acts only on diseased organs having pathological symptoms. And in proving the drug, he writes that homeopathic drugs produce symptoms in healthy organs of the healthy body when given in 30th potency, a very minute quantity of drug. Again this is a contradiction. If homeopathic drugs produce symptoms in healthy organs of healthy human beings, then they might produce symptoms in healthy organs of patients. But he refused it.

At one point Hahnemann writes that after the removal of natural disease, remaining morbid symptoms of drug in the body "disappear so rapidly of its own accord that the vital force has no need to employ" (Hahnemann, 1921/1993, p. 153) and when natural disease has been removed, vital force does not require to do any effort to abolish remaining drug-induced symptoms (Hahnemann, 1921/1996, p. 91).

At another point he writes that after removal of natural disease, drug-induced symptoms of short duration are abolished by vital force (Hahnemann, 1921/1996, p. 49) and "In the homeopathic curative operation the living organism reacts from these only so much as it requisite to raise the health again to the normal healthy state" (Hahnemann, 1921/1993, p. 193) and vital force uses its power against the drug-induced effect (Hahnemann, 1921/1996, p. 85), which indicates that Hahnemann himself was not clear. There are many contradictions in explanations given by him.

Hahnemann said that if symptoms produced by drugs are more powerful and stronger than similar symptoms of disease, then only cure is possible, because powerful and strong symptoms of drugs only replace comparatively weaker and similar symptoms of disease. This indicates that a patient suffering from pain in abdomen can get cured only by that homeopathic drug which can create more severe pain in abdomen. If a homeopathic drug develops a more intense headache in a patient who is suffering from a headache, then only the drug will be effective. It cannot be possible for a drug to cure a disease by producing pathology in the same organ as produced by disease itself. It will rather aggravate the problem. Hahnemann said that homeopathic drugs have no effect on healthy organs. It acts only on diseased organs having pathological symptoms.

References

Ganong, W. F. (2003). *Review of medical physiology* (22nd ed.). Boston, MA: McGraw Hill.

Hahnemann, S. (1993). *Organon of medicine* (6th ed.) (W. Boericke, Trans.). New Delhi, India: B. Jain Publishers. (Original work published in 1921).

Hahnemann, S. (1996). *Organon of medicine* (6th ed.) (P. Devi, Trans.). New Delhi, India: B. Jain Publishers. (Original work published in 1921).

Hahnemann, S. (2017). *Organon of medicine* (6th ed.) (W. Boericke, Trans). New Delhi, India: B. Jain Publishers. (Original work published in 1921).

Satoskar, R. S. & Bhandarkar, S. D. (1988). *Pharmacology and pharmacotherapeutics* (11th ed.). Mumbai, India: Elsevier and Popular Prakashan.

Vaz, M. (2016). General physiology: Functional organization of the human body and control of the internal environment. In J. E. Hall, M. Viz, A. Kurpad, & T. Raj (Eds.), *Guyton and Hall textbook of medical physiology* (Second South Asia Edition, pp. 3–8). Delhi, India: Elsevier (RELX India Pvt. Ltd).

chapter sixteen

Mercuric chloride and syphilis

Basic concept of homeopathy – sixteen

According to the rules of homeopathy, mercuric chloride is effective in very dilute concentration and its toxic effect is similar to symptomatology of syphilis.

Argument

Hahnemann made an important law of homeopathy "Like cures like", by observation of cinchona and mercury. Cinchona was used in malaria and mercury was used in syphilis.

"Hahnemann had been impressed with the particular symptoms which mercury could produce and had associated these with its healing capacities in syphilis" (Hobhouse, 1984, p. 78). Because of this his conclusion was displacing a disease by a medicine which could cause similar states to those which it could cure (Hobhouse, 1984).

It has already been explained earlier how Hahnemann concluded wrongly by observing the cinchona effect in malaria and in healthy human beings. Now it is being explained how Hahnemann was misled by mercury.

> Many chemicals are toxic to cell protoplasm. In certain instances they may possess a specific affinity and toxicity for micro-organisms of a special type e.g., antimalarial drugs. In other cases the effect upon cells may be nonselective and cells of the host as well as invading bacteria may be killed. Protoplasmic poison (mercury salts and silver salts) belong to the latter category. For this reason these agents must be used judiciously as antiseptic. (Krantz & Carr, 1965, pp. 205–206)

"The metal acts in extremely low concentration if allowed sufficient time. Mercuric chloride kills *B. Typhosus* at dilution of 1 in 1000000 in 24 hours and at a dilution of 1 in 20000 in 22 minutes" (Wilson et al., 1975, p. 550). "Mercury was the first drug effective in treatment of syphilis" (Wilson et al., 1975, p. 234). "Like other mercury salts mercuric chloride has a specific toxic action against *Treponema pallidum* and has been used in treatment of syphilis" (Wilson et al., 1975, p. 234). Mercury is highly toxic to the body, 1–5 µg/ml concentration of mercury in blood produces various toxic manifestations. Acute mercury poisoning is characterized by ashen gray appearance of the mouth, pharynx, and gastric mucosa, vomiting, diarrhea, emphysema, hemorrhage. Kidney, colon, and month are also affected. Renal lesions are also produced. In chronic mercury poisoning, features are paresthesias, ataxia, visual defects, dysarthria, hearing defects, tremors, and various neurological and psychiatric symptoms. Irritability, erethism, insomnia, confusion, and forgetfulness are common psychiatric symptoms of chronic mercury poisoning. Nephrotoxicity, gingivitis, stomatitis, and other nonspecific symptoms such as anorexia, weight loss, anemia, and weakness are also associated with chronic mercury poisoning (Klaassen, 1980, pp. 1623–1625).

The symptomatology of syphilis is more or less akin to mercury toxic manifestations. Syphilis is a chronic systemic infection caused by *Treponema pallidum*, a spirochete (a microorganism). Syphilis has wide symptomatology. These are macular, papular, papulosquamous skin rashes; mucosa erosions in lips, oral mucosa, tongue, palate, pharynx, vulva, vagina; silver-gray erosive mucosa patches surrounded by red periphery; fever, weight loss, malaise, anorexia, gastritis, hepatitis, nephropathy, arthritis, ocular disturbances, optic neuritis, ataxia, paresthesias, bladder disturbances, abnormalities regarding personality, illusion, delusion, hallucination, alteration on intellect functions. Renal involvement is associated with proteinuria, an acute nephritic syndrome or with hemorrhage (Holmes, 1983, pp. 1034–1040).

By observing and comparing mercury toxicity and syphilis manifestation, we can say that both are more or less similar. But with this similarity, "the rule", like cures like, cannot be formulated. The observation of Hahnemann was correct but the conclusion was wrong. Why?

> Mercury and its compounds are absorbed through the skin by ingestion and by inhalation. Inorganic compounds of mercury are absorbed through the gastrointestinal tract better than the organic compounds of mercury ... Mercurous compounds and metallic mercury are oxidized and the mercury salts form soluble compounds with proteins, sodium chloride, blood and tissue fluid alkalis ... Mercury inhibits enzyme systems and disturbs mitochondrial functions. Mercury also combines

Chapter sixteen: Mercuric chloride and syphilis 53

with sulfhydryl and phosphoryl groups in the cell membrane. (Hennigar, 1971, pp. 209–212)

Infection in syphilis occurs by penetration of the spirochetes through a microscopic break in the epithelial lining of the mucosa or the skin into connective tissue. There they rapidly multiply, penetrate the lymphatics and invade the bloodstream producing a systemic spirochetemia … This organism may produce extensive tissue necrosis involving all tissues of the body. (Haam, 1971, pp. 350–352)

Mercury produces various toxic manifestations because it damages cells and ultimately tissues of various organs of the body. Spirochete, a causative organism in syphilis, also produces more or less similar symptomatology because it also damages various organs of the body. Mercury has nonspecific action, it destroys human cells as well as foreign microorganisms, which may be spirochaetes or bacteria. The concentration of mercury, which is required to kill spirochetes, also destroys the human cells. Mercury also destroys bacteria and it is also effective as an antibacterial and antiseptic. In various bacterial infections, mercury is effective but these bacterial infections such as *Bacillus typhosus* never produce symptomatology like mercury-toxic manifestations. This finding is against the law discovered by Hahnemann. Mercury is effective in very low concentration. This misled Hahnemann that all drugs could be effective in very low concentration.

This happens by chance that mercury and *T. pallidum* both have common pathogenesis for producing toxic effects in the human body. But by this observation, generalization cannot be made. Nowadays, mercury is not used in systemic infections due to its toxic manifestations. Penicillin is the drug of choice for syphilis. When penicillin is administered in healthy human beings, it never produces syphilis like symptomatology. It again opposes the Hahnemann law.

References

Haam, E. V. (1971). Venereal diseases and spirochetal infections. In W. A. D. Anderson (Ed.), *Pathology* (6th ed., Vol. 1, pp. 341–364). St. Louis, MO: C.V. Mosby Company.

Hennigar, G. R. (1971). Effect of radiation. In W. A. D. Anderson (Ed.), *Pathology* (6th ed., Vol. 1, pp. 174–241). St. Louis, MO: C.V. Mosby Company.

Hobhouse, R. W. (1984). *Life of Christian Samuel Hahnemann*. New Delhi, India: World Homeopathic Links.

Holmes, K. K. (1983). Syphilis. In R. G. Petersdorf, R. D. Adams, E. Braunwald, K. J. Isselbacher, J. B. Martin, & J. D. Wilson (Eds.), *Harrison's principle of internal medicine* (10th ed., pp. 1034–1045). New Delhi, India: McGraw Hill.

Klaassen, C. D. (1980). Heavy metals and heavy metals antagonists. In A. G. Gilman, L. Goodman, & A. Gilman (Eds.), *Goodman and Gilman's pharmacological basis of therapeutics* (6th ed., pp. 1615–1637). New York, NY: Macmillan.

Krantz, J. C., & Carr, C. J. (1965). *The pharmacological principles of medical practice* (Indian 6th ed.). Baltimore, MD: Williams and Wilkins Company.

Wilson, A., Schild, H. O., & Modell, W. (1975). *Applied pharmacology* (11th ed.). London, United Kingdom: ELBS & Churchill Livingstone.

chapter seventeen

Effect of opium

Basic concept of homeopathy – seventeen

Hahnemann observed the effect of opium on human beings and found two types of effects: direct and indirect. Both were opposite to each other. He said that the first direct action was the initial aggravation of symptoms. A similar effect was also found when sulfur had been given to treat skin diseases.

Argument

Hahnemann observed in his practice that medicine has two types of effects, direct and indirect. He gives an example of opium. "This drug at first produces a fearless elevation of spirit, a sensation of strength and high courage, an imaginative gaiety. But after some hours have passed we find the person so elevated as a first result of taking the drug relaxed, dejected, peevish with confused memory and generally discomforted and fearful" (Hobhouse, 1984, p. 131). First action is a direct action and secondary action is an indirect action. "Hahnemann welcomed the first action, some accentuation of the patient's symptoms. The secondary or indirect action decided in favour of reduction in the symptoms and in cure" (Hobhouse, 1984, p. 131).

Initial aggravation of symptoms by opium was called the first action of the drug, and on the basis of this concept Hahnemann made another concept of homeopathy. By this observation, Hahnemann made another false concept of homeopathy as he writes, "The slight homeopathic aggravation during the first hours – a very good prognostic that the acute disease will most probably yield to the first dose – is quite as it ought to be" (Hahnemann, 2017, p. 161).

Cause of this aggravation was given by Hahnemann as follow:

> Immediately after ingestion – for the first hour or for a few hours causes a kind of slight aggravation when the dose as not be in sufficiently small which has so much resemblance to the original disease that it seems to the patient to be an aggravation of his own disease. But it is in reality nothing more

DOI: 10.1201/9781003228622-17

55

than an extremely similar medicinal disease, somewhat exceeding in strength the original affection.
(Hahnemann, 2017, p. 161)

Hahnemann suggested that this aggravation of symptoms is due to similar symptomatology produced by drugs as well as symptoms produced by disease. This suggestion was made on the basis of the effects produced by opium in a healthy body. Here Hahnemann once again made the wrong conclusion. How? Opium and its derivatives are drugs of addiction. Morphine (opium derivatives) produces a sense of emotional well-being termed as euphoria. Euphoria eliminates the normal fear, panic, and aids the analgesic action of morphine. The ability to produce euphoria makes morphine one of the worst drugs of addiction (Satoskar & Bhandarkar, 1988, p. 121).

The euphoric effect produced by opium confused Hahnemann who later framed the wrong homeopathic concept of aggravation of symptoms by homeopathic drugs. Euphoria means false sense of well-being which is produced by opium. This effect confused Hahnemann and he correlated this euphoric effect with aggravation of disease symptoms wrongly. I am writing again and again that single or few observations do not make any conclusion. There should be a controlled experiment that must be done by a good expert, and then only the conclusion can be drawn.

The exaltation of the medicinal symptoms is also observed by other physicians who accidently prescribed homeopathic remedy. "When a patient suffering from itch complains so an increase of the eruption after sulfur, his physician who knows not the cause of this consoles him with the assurance that the itch must first come out properly before it can be cured" (Hahnemann, 1993, pp. 221–222).

Sulfur is applied to the skin for skin infection. Sulfur is converted into pentathionic acid that exerted germicidal action. Sulfur also possesses a keratolytic property that may be the basis for the therapeutic action in certain skin diseases. Sulfur is used as a fungicide and parasiticide. It is used in the treatment of skin disorders such as psoriasis, seborrhea, and dermatitis. Prolong local use of sulfur may result in characteristic dermatitis (Harvey, 1980, pp. 980–981). It is an acute allergic inflammation of the skin caused by contact with sulfur.

Again we can conclude that exaltation of itch is actually sulfur eruption that assumes the appearance of an increase of the itch. This fact was not known to these physicians, because of that they arrived at the wrong conclusion and made the wrong generalization. These actions of opium and sulfur are very specific and on the basis of this concept the general rule cannot be made.

Chapter seventeen: Effect of opium   57

References

Hahnemann, S. (1993). *Organon of medicine* (6th ed.) (W. Boericke, Trans.). New Delhi, India: B. Jain Publishers. (Original work published in 1921).

Hahnemann, S. (2017). *Organon of medicine* (6th ed.) (W. Boericke, Trans.). New Delhi, India: B. Jain Publishers (P) Ltd. (Original work published in 1921).

Harvey, S. C. (1980). Antiseptic and disinfectants; fungicides; ectoparasiticided. In A. G. Gilman, L. Goodman, & A. Gilman (Eds.), *Goodman and Gilman's pharmacological basis of therapeutics* (6th ed., pp. 964–987). New York, NY: Macmillan.

Hobhouse, R. W. (1984). *Life of Christian Samuel Hahnemann*. New Delhi, India: World Homeopathic Links.

Satoskar, R. S., & Bhandarkar, S. D. (1988). *Pharmacology and pharmacotherapeutics* (11th ed.). Bombay, India: Popular Prakashan.

chapter eighteen

Manic episode

Basic concept of homeopathy – eighteen

About the year 1500, Melampus, a most celebrated physician, cured the daughters of Proteus, who were affected by wandering mania; they were cured chiefly by means of veratrum album. As the plant could also cause mania, the story was of twofold interest to Hahnemann.

Argument

In support of Hahnemann's law of similarity, examples were given from history.

> About the year 1500, Melampus ... a most celebrated physician cured the daughters of Proteus, who were affected by a wandering mania, they were cured chiefly by means of veratrum album, given in the milk of goats fed upon veratrum. As the plant could also cause mania, the story was of too fold interest to Hahnemann. (Hobhouse, 1984, pp. 135–136)

In this example, two things are important. First, veratrum cured mania, and second, veratrum produced mania. This example supported Hahnemann's law of similarity.

To assess the effect of a drug, we should know what the normal course of a disease is when we are not giving any treatment. Knowledge of the natural course of a disease is very important in the absence of treatment. To study the effect of a drug, two groups of patients are usually made. Each group consists of a large number of patients according to study material. Drugs are given to one group. For the second group, an inert material is given for the treatment to see the placebo (psychological) effect. On the basis of statistical analysis, conclusions can be drawn. Observing only one or few patients, without a systematic controlled study, nothing can be concluded.

If we find that in the natural course, without taking any drug, a disease subsides automatically, then how can we say that disease is cured by taking a drug. For example, bacillary dysentery is cured automatically

DOI: 10.1201/9781003228622-18

within 24 hours without taking any treatment. If we give any treatment to this patient, it will seem to be effective. But it will not be the truth. It will be a false conclusion. Similarly, manic episodes subside automatically, and after a period of normality, again there is an episode of the manic reaction. It is a normal cycle for manic patients that first mania then normality, and after some time, there is again mania.

Manic depressive reactions are episodic and brief. Even without treatment, manic and depressive reactions usually run their course in about three to nine months. There are wide variations also. At the end of an episode, the individual usually returns to apparent normality (Coleman, 1976, p. 341).

It is also mentioned in psychiatry,

> Duration of episodes in the predrug era averaged about one year for depression and four months for mania ... Patients who present with only symptoms of depression take almost twice as long to recover from their episode (a median of 9 weeks) as do patients present with only symptoms of mania (a median of 5 weeks) ... Short term recovery rates also differ among subtypes ... Bipolar patients however are more likely than unipolar patients to have multiple subsequent episodes. (Hirschfeld & Goodwin, 1988, p. 414)

From the above discussion, we can conclude that in manic patients, Hahnemann wrongly observed that by giving veratrum, patients are improving, and by giving veratrum, patients get an attack of mania. The second point in favor of our argument is that veratrum alkaloid does not produce any psychological and neurological effects when given to healthy persons. Hahnemann observed an attack of mania in these patients after giving veratrum, who were already suffering from mania. Once a patient has suffered from mania, there are chances that he will again get an episode of mania. It is a normal cycle. He concluded wrongly that it was veratrum that is responsible for recurrence of manic episodes. Veratrum has no psychological effect. Protoveratrine A and B, alkaloids of veratrum, "on oral administration 1 to 25 mg daily in divided doses is effective in lowering the blood pressure in about 1/3 of the patients with hypertension. Unless dosage is regulated carefully toxic effects such as nausea, vomiting, hiccough, severe hypotension, bradycardia or even heart block appear" (Krantz & Carr, 1965, p. 692). Veratrum does not cause mania or depression.

Chapter eighteen: Manic episode   61

References

Coleman, J. (1976). *Abnormal psychology and modern life.* Bombay, India: Taraporewala and Sons.

Hirschfeld, R. M. A., & Goodwin, F. K. (1988). Mood disorders. In J. A. Talbot, R. E. Hales, & S. C. Yudofsky (Eds.), *Textbook of psychiatry* (pp. 403–441). Washington, WA: American Psychiatric press.

Hobhouse, R. W. (1984). *Life of Christian Samuel Hahnemann.* New Delhi, India: World Homeopathic Links.

Krantz, J. C., & Carr, C. J. (1965). *The pharmacological principles of medical practice* (Indian 6th ed.). Baltimore, MD: Williams and Wilkins Company.

chapter nineteen

Scarlet fever and belladonna

Basic concept of homeopathy – nineteen

Hahneman recommended belladonna for the treatment of scarlet fever in an infinitesimal dose because it produces fever. In 1838, the Prussian government ordered doctors to use belladonna in small doses against the epidemics of scarlet fever because it was effective. It supported Hahnemann's law, "like cures like".

Argument

Treatment of scarlet fever by belladonna also created confusion in the mind of Hahnemann. Hahnemann used belladonna for scarlet fever because it produces fever. This medicine he administered in a very high potency, which is in an infinitesimal dose (Hobhouse, 1984, pp. 142–143).

Hahnemann writes,

> Furnished me with no remedy so capable of producing a counterpart if the symptoms here present as belladonna. I, therefore, gave this girl of ten years of age, who was already affected by the first stages of scarlet fever, a dose of this medicine 1/432999th of a grain of the extract, which according to my subsequent experience is rather too large a dose. So remarkable was the effect that the following day she was playing again, complaining of nothing and quite lively. (Hobhouse, 1984, p. 143)

This observation compelled Hahnemann to think regarding the preventive aspect of belladonna in scarlet fever.

> The doctor then recollected that some weeks previously he had visited a family where three children lay sick with scarlet fever, the eldest daughter alone, who had been taking belladonna ... not having sickened. And this though during previous epidemics the eldest daughter had shown a disposition to take

DOI: 10.1201/9781003228622-19

then first. He straightway, therefore gave to the remaining five children of the family he was now attending very small doses of the drug every seventy two hours and they all remained well throughout the epidemics. (Hobhouse, 1984, p. 143)

"In 1838 Prussian Government ordered the doctors of the country to use belladonna in small doses against the epidemics of scarlet fever" (Hobhouse, 1984, p. 145). However some physicians had opposed the Hahnemann by saying about "smallness of the dose". It was also stated that powder contained no belladonna. But it had been established at that time the belladonna was effective in scarlet fever, as a curative and a preventive drug.

Now we are analyzing treatment of scarlet fever by belladonna. Belladonna produces fever in healthy individuals and it is effective in scarlet fever as told by Hahnemann and which also supported a law of similarity, framed by Hahnemann. Today we know that belladonna drugs are widely distributed in nature, especially in the solanaceae plants. Atropa belladonna yields mainly the alkaloid atropine.

The rise in body temperature due to the belladonna alkaloids is usually significant only after large doses. Nevertheless in infants and small children moderate doses induce atropine fever ... Suppression of sweating is doubtless a considerable factor in the production of the fever ... Animals that do not sweat such as the dog do not exhibit fever after atropine. (Weiner, 1980, p. 126)

The observation of Hahnemann that belladonna causes an increase in body temperature was correct. Today we know the mechanism by which belladonna increases body temperature. Suppression of sweating is mainly responsible for pyrexia. The second part of this observation that belladonna is effective in scarlet fever was wrong.

It became apparent that only a minority of adults were susceptible to scarlet fever and that the number who were immune was far in excess of the number who had actually had the disease previously ... It appears that repeated experiences with streptococcus pyogenes may confer immunity to scarlet fever even though the disease, per se, has not been experienced ... The importance of individual variation

Chapter nineteen: Scarlet fever and belladonna 65

> in the host is illustrated by the fact that several or all members of a family may develop streptococcal pharyngitis from the same strain of organism, yet only one of the group may develop scarlet fever the other manifesting only nasopharyngitis. (Hoppes, 1971, p. 287)

If microorganism is virulent and size of the infecting dose is high, the disease will be severe and in opposite conditions, disease will be mild. Similarly, host resistance also plays an important role. If host resistance is high, disease will be mild, and if host resistance is poor, disease will be severe. This rule is true for all bacterial, viral, and other infections "Variations in host resistance are often the result of variation in the host's ability to form antibodies" (Hoppes, 1971, p. 274). Now we can conclude that the intensity of scarlet fever will be mild if host resistance is high or the infecting organism has low virulence and low doses.

During observation of scarlet fever it has been found that,

> Scarlet fever has many varieties. In the mild type the patient never appears particularly ill. Toxaemia is negligible, the temperature does not exceed 38.30°C (101°F) and symptomatic recovery takes place within 3 to 4 days. This type of scarlet fever covers a larger percentage of cases. In the more severe cases the prodromal symptoms are more striking with the temperature reaching 104°F, the rash heavier and lasting for a few days while fever and constitutional symptoms may persist up to a week. Complications are more common to this group. (McKendrick, 1978, p. 67)

Now we can understand very well where Hahnemann committed the mistake.

Hahnemann cured a patient of scarlet fever, who had been suffering from the first stage of scarlet fever. Actually this patient had been suffering from mild scarlet fever. The cure was automatic and mild scarlet fever has a very short course. During automatic recovery of mild scarlet fever, Hahnemann administered belladonna and concluded wrongly that cure was due to belladonna. Hahnemann did not know that the mild type of scarlet fever recovers early. It has been mentioned that the eldest daughter who had been taking belladonna did not suffer from scarlet fever and he also mentioned that this eldest daughter had suffered from scarlet fever in previous years. Today we know that if a person suffers from scarlet fever, he develops immunity to scarlet fever and then he will never develop this disease in future infections. This fact was not known previously. That's why he derived the wrong conclusion. He did not understand that once this elder daughter suffered from scarlet fever. She should not have suffered from scarlet fever in the coming years due to immunity. The immunity of the eldest daughter to scarlet fever was not related to belladonna in any way.

Hahnemann has mentioned that children who were taking belladonna did not suffer from scarlet fever because of belladonna. It is also wrong. We know by the present study that it is not necessary that all members of family should suffer from scarlet fever during epidemics. Some may suffer from pharyngitis only to give immunity to scarlet fever. It has been found during epidemics that only a few members of the family suffered from scarlet fever, rest of the members remain healthy without giving belladonna or any other treatment. So this is the truth that belladonna has no preventive and curative role in scarlet fever. Again this origin of the homeopathic concept is wrong.

References

Hobhouse, R. W. (1984). *Life of Christian Samuel Hahnemann*. New Delhi, India: World Homeopathic Links.

Hoppes, H. C. (1971). Bacterial diseases. In W. A. D. Anderson (Ed.), *Pathology* (6th ed., Vol. 1, pp. 270–327). St. Louis, MO: C.V. Mosby Company.

McKendrick, G. D. W. (1978). Scarlet fever. In R. B. Scott (Ed.), *Price's textbook of the practice of medicine* (12th ed., pp. 65–68). Oxford, United Kingdom: ELBS and Oxford University Press.

Weiner, N. (1980). Atropine, scopolamine, and related antimuscarinic drugs. In A. G. Gilman, L. Goodman, & A. Gilman (Eds.), *Goodman and Gilman's pharmacological basis of therapeutics* (6th ed., pp. 120–137). New York, NY: Macmillan.

chapter twenty

Grinding gives power and color

Basic concept of homeopathy – twenty

Clinical experience proved that the medicinal virtues were undoubtedly increased by the process of attenuation, trituration, and succussion. By dilution and trituration, effects of mercury and arsenic are increased. Upon grinding, insoluble substances become soluble and give colors, which also supports the view that dilution increases power.

Argument

One of the main concepts of homeopathy is potentization, which means increased potency by dilution and trituration. Homeopaths say, "As clinical experience proved that the medicinal virtues were undoubtedly increased by the process of attenuation, trituration and succussion, Hahnemann called those process potentisation, that is a making more potent for cure though less powerful for harm" (Hobhouse, 1984, p. 146).

Hahnemann also wrote,

> Pure gold, silver, platinum have no action on the health in their solid state-nor crude vegetable, charcoal etc. These substances are in a state of suspended animation as regards the medicinal action, but triturate one grain of gold leaf with 100 grains of sugar of milk and a preparation results which has already great medicinal power. (Hobhouse, 1984, p. 146)

The dilution and trituration effects of mercury are increased. But this potentization is not due to dilute mercury, but it is due to the formation of mercuric oxide, which is highly potent in higher dilution than concentrated mercury. With the knowledge of chemistry, we know that "Silver undergoes no change in water or pure air. Silver is unaffected by caustic alkalis even on fusion and by vegetable acids. Dilute hydrochloric acid and sulfuric acid also have no action" (Soni, 1981, p. 2.141). "Gold does not tarnish when exposed to air or oxygen even at high temperature. Common acids do not attack it if used singly" (Soni, 1981, p. 2.154). "Platinum is a noble metal and is very slightly affected even on prolonged heating in air.

It is very resistant to the action or acids. Boiling concentrated sulfuric acid attacks it to a slight extent" (Soni, 1981, p. 3.311).

The above given information from various studies (Soni, 1981) shows that metals such as silver, gold, and platinum after dilution and trituration do not modify into other compounds because these are highly resistant to air, water, and acid. While mercury and arsenic change into other compounds after trituration and dilution, which are highly potent than original metals. As we know about arsenic from the study that

> Metallic arsenic is not poisonous as it is insoluble in water and therefore incapable of absorption from the alimentary canal but it oxidizes by exposure to the air and then becomes poisonous. It is believed that some portion of elementary arsenic may undergo oxidation in the alimentary canal under some conditions that may produce poisonous symptoms. (Modi, 1975, p. 521)

As we also know from the study that "when arsenic is burnt in air, arsenious oxide is produced which acts as a violent irritant poison" (Soni, 1981, pp. 3.95 and 3.96).

With the help of above information, we can conclude that mercury and arsenic gave wrong impressions to Hahnemann. Hahnemann concluded wrongly about mercury and arsenic. Mercury and arsenic in their original metallic forms were not potent, but after dilution and trituration both were converted into other compounds, which are potent and toxic in dilute forms and effective in some disease, but they are highly toxic. Hahnemann's conclusions regarding silver, gold, and platinum were also wrong. These metals after dilution and trituration never become potent. They are not effective in medicine in their original metallic forms. These metals in high dilution have no effect on any disease.

Today mercury and arsenic are not used as a drug because these are highly toxic even in high dilutions. But mercury and arsenic give the wrong foundation to homeopathy because these metals, after dilution and trituration, are converted into potent compounds. These observations made the wrong law of homeopathy that dilution and trituration increased potency of a substance. Supporters of homeopathy also give examples of colloids by mistake. They believed that insoluble substances on grinding become soluble and give colors. These colors represent the hidden power of substances. It has been said that by grinding, insoluble substances became soluble, which represents an increase in their medicinal power. Hahnemann supported this concept and stated that "Grinding

Chapter twenty: Grinding gives power and color 69

of gold for medicinal purposes finely enough to pass into something approaching a soluble state" (Hobhouse, 1984, p. 150).

Homeopaths took the support of Cennino.

> Cennino left his directions for the preparation of vegetable and mineral substances for use in painting of pictures explaining how by various degrees of pulverisation their peculiar beauties could be released of the blue made from grinding lapis lazuli to a powder. Cennino speaks as noble, beautiful and perfect beyond all other colours. (Hobhouse, 1984, p. 150)

"By grinding insoluble substances become soluble and give colours. It is due to formation of colloids" (Soni, 1981, p. 2.82).

If sand is shaken with water, a suspension results. Because of the large size of the sand particles they would settle down on standing. If particle size is reduced gradually, then at the size of 1–100 nm a colloidal state is formed. In this condition, the solution appears homogeneous and particles do not settle down on standing. Particles are not separable by filtration. Coarser particles are broken to the colloidal size by grinding and the color of the colloidal solution depends upon (a) size and shape of particles, (b) wavelength of the light falling on solution, (c) selective absorption power of solution, (d) observer receives the light by transmission or reflection. Conclusively, it can be said that the colloidal state does not indicate a class of substances but is a state. Any substance can be brought into the colloidal state.

Hahnemann did not know about colloids, that's why he wrongly interpreted this state. Not only gold but any substance can also be transformed into the colloidal state. In this state, the substance gives color and becomes soluble. This state depends on particle size and does not give any extra medicinal capacity to that substance.

References

Hobhouse, R. W. (1984). *Life of Christian Samuel Hahnemann*. New Delhi, India: World Homeopathic Links.

Modi, N. J. (1975). *Textbook of medical jurisprudence and toxicology* (9th ed.). Bombay, India: N.M. Tripathi, Publisher.

Soni, P. L. (1981). *Textbook of inorganic chemistry* (13th ed.). New Delhi, India: Sultan Chand and Sons Publications.

chapter twenty one

Treatment of cholera

Basic concept of homeopathy – twenty one

Allopathic treatment was unscientific, wrong, and responsible for more harm than cure. Hahnemann opposed allopathy and established homeopathy. One prescription of Hahnemann which made him very popular was treatment of cholera. Allopathy was not able to cure the patients of cholera but homeopathy did it.

Argument

I am saying repeatedly that allopathic treatment prevalent at the time of Hahnemann was unscientific, wrong, and responsible for more harm than cure. That treatment was completely different from allopathy of the present day, which is absolutely scientific and based on practical knowledge.

Here is one more example of old allopathic treatment. "Nervous attacks from early childhood were treated by MOXA and trephine. Moxa is a cylinder of readily combustible material which is burnt on the skin. Trephine means removal of a part of the bone of the skull" (Hobhouse, 1984, p. 241). Old allopathic treatment of Hahnemann's time was harmful. Homeopathic treatment was actually no treatment. No treatment is always better than harmful treatment. Harmful treatment damages the body, while no treatment does not interfere with the immunity of the body, which is helpful in fighting the disease.

One more example has been given here.

One doctor,

> Lagusius had admittedly tried to fight the severe fever and its accompanying symptoms by venesection and when this failed to give relief he proceeded to open the veins again and yet again until blood-letting had been resorted to for a fourth time … To abstract the fluid of life four times in twenty four hours from a man who has lost flesh from mental overwork combined with a long continued diarrhoea without procuring any improvement. (Hobhouse, 1984, pp. 82–83)

DOI: 10.1201/9781003228622-21

72 *Homeopathy*

One prescription of Hahnemann which made him very popular was treatment of cholera. In this prescription, camphor was directed to the arresting of cholera.

> Hahnemann had not treated or even seen one single cholera patient. Hahnemann had procured a very accurate description of the symptoms and had found that the first and most important of these in cholera patient resembled one another and were similar to the symptoms produced if camphor was taken in large quantities by a healthy individual. (Hobhouse, 1984, p. 242)

When camphor is given in large amounts, it produces symptomatology similar to cholera because camphor is an irritant substance to the gastrointestinal tract.

> Hahnemann had, therefore, concluded from the great similarity of the symptoms at the beginning of the disease with those brought out by camphor in proving that this ought to be the best remedy to give at the outset. In the similar way he also prescribed the other remedies required for the cure of the later stages of cholera. (Hobhouse, 1984, p. 242)

According to Hahnemann at the early stage of cholera, camphor in high dilution is effective, but in the later stage of cholera, other drugs are effective. Using this treatment Hahnemann had become very popular. "In 1854 a report to the House of Commons gave the figures of death from cholera under orthodox treatment at 59.2 percent and under the homeopathic treatment at 16.4 percent. In all 54000 persons died" (Hobhouse, 1984, p. 249).

With the success of the cholera treatment homeopathy became very popular throughout the world. But it was the wrong popularity of homeopathic treatment. I am describing the fact here. Cholera is an acute diarrheal disease caused by *Vibrio cholerae*. Studies have shown that more than 90% of cholera cases are mild. In severe cases of cholera, painless watery diarrhea is followed by vomiting. The patient soon reaches a stage of collapse because of dehydration. Death may occur at this stage due to dehydration and acidosis. If death does not occur, the patient begins to show signs of improvement. The classical form of severe cholera occurs in only

Chapter twenty one: Treatment of cholera 73

5–10% of cases. In the rest the disease tends to be mild, characterized by diarrhea with or without vomiting. Generally, mild cases recover in one to three days (Park, 1997, pp. 163–170).

When the treatment of cholera is considered, it is mentioned clearly in modern medical science, "The disease runs its course in 2 to 7 days and subsequent manifestations depend on the adequacy of electrolyte repletion therapy. With prompt fluid and electrolyte repletion, physiological recovery is remarkably rapid and mortality exceptionally rare" (Carpenter, 1983, p. 997).

Now we compare homeopathic treatment of cholera, old allopathic orthodox treatment, and modern medical treatment. With the help of modern medical treatment, the death rate in cholera is zero. There is no death if modern medical treatment is given. This indicates there is a 100% cure rate by modern medical treatment. We also know that 90% cholera cases are mild and recover automatically within one to three days. There is a 10% death rate in cholera if no treatment is given. When homeopathic treatment is given, there is a death rate of 16.4%. Death rate during homeopathic treatment is the same as when any type of treatment is not given. This indicates homeopathy treatment is equal to no treatment in cholera patients.

When orthodox old allopathic treatment is given in cholera, there is a death rate of 59.2%. When treatment is not given, there is a death rate of 10% only. This suggests that there is a damaging influence of old orthodox treatment in cholera, and this is correct.

> Medicine as commonly practiced in allopathy knows no treatment except to draw from diseases the injurious materials which are assumed to be their cause. The blood of the patient is made to flow, mercilessly by bleeding ... medicine as commonly practised seeks to evacuate the contents of the stomach and sweep the intestine clear of the materials assumed to originate diseases. (Hahnemann, 1921/1993, p. 15)

Medicine employed in cholera in orthodox allopathic treatment increases blood and water loss. Cholera causes water loss which is further increased by old allopathic treatment. That's why there is an increased death rate with old allopathic treatment. Now we can conclude that old allopathic treatment of cholera is the worst, homeopathic treatment is no treatment, while modern medical treatment is accurate and gives a 100% cure rate.

References

Carpenter, C. C. J. (1983). Cholera. In R. G. Petersdorf, R. D. Adams, E. Braunwald, K. J. Isselbacher, J. B. Martin, & J. D. Wilson (Eds.), *Harrison's principle of internal medicine* (10th ed., pp. 996–998). New Delhi, India: McGraw Hill.

Hahnemann, S. (1993). *Organon of medicine* (6th ed.) (W. Boericke, Trans.). New Delhi, India: B. Jain Publishers. (Original work published in 1921).

Hobhouse, R. W. (1984). *Life of Christian Samuel Hahnemann*. New Delhi, India: World Homeopathic Links.

Park, K. (1997). *Park's textbook of preventive and social medicine* (15th ed.). Jabalpur, India: Banarsidas Bhanot Publisher.

chapter twenty two

Psora

Basic concept of homeopathy – twenty two

According to homeopathy, the cause of diseases is actually inside the body not outside. Bacteria, viruses, protozoa, mosquitoes, dirty water, unhygienic food, and pollution are not responsible for any disease. The basic cause of all diseases is psora and that is developed due to wrong assumption. Sinful thoughts and acts are responsible for all chronic diseases. If a person has pure thoughts in his mind, he/she cannot suffer from any disease.

Argument

Homeopathy says, it is useless to spend money in finding the cause of diseases. The government is spending lakhs of rupees unnecessarily in such studies. Why this truth cannot be accepted by people that the cause of diseases is actually inside the body and not outside the body (Ghatak, 1931/1938, pp. 1–2).

Do you accept this statement of homeopathy? The development of medical science is not only dependent on medical research but is also related to the total development of science. Invention of microscope in physics is responsible for discovery of bacteria and viruses. In the absence of a microscope, it was not possible to search for bacteria and viruses. Discovery of bacteria and viruses indicated that these organisms are responsible for diseases, which gives tremendous help to medical science. Medical science also takes help from physics, chemistry, botany, zoology, biotechnology, and genetics. Concepts of medical science are based on various branches of science. As we know, today, that malaria is a protozoal disease caused by parasites of the genus *Plasmodium* and transmitted to human beings by certain species of infected female, Anopheles mosquito. Ronald Ross discovered the transmission of malaria by an Anopheles mosquito in 1897. Ross found malarial parasites growing as a cyst on the stomach wall of an Anopheles mosquito. Upon killing of mosquitoes by D.D.T. and destroying malarial parasites by antimalarial drugs, malaria came down to extremely low levels. We all know these facts, but how can we accept this concept of homeopathy that malaria is not caused by malarial parasites? Similarly in homeopathy, killing of parasites and mosquitoes are not required in treatment of malaria.

DOI: 10.1201/9781003228622-22

According to homeopathy, the basic cause of all diseases is psora. If there is no psora in the body, there cannot be any disease. Psora is developed due to wrong assumption and can transfer from generation to generation (Ghatak, 1931/1938, pp. 4–7). Moreover, psora expresses itself by skin disease associated with itching. According to this concept, cancer, cardiovascular problems, joint problems, dysentery, malaria, typhoid, gall stone, hemiplegia, tuberculosis, leprosy, polio, cholera, and all other diseases are due to psora, which is originated due to wrong thoughts.

Homeopathy also says, psora is the result of sinful thought, while sycosis and syphilis are the result of sinful acts. Without psora, sycosis and syphilis cannot be developed. These three are responsible for all chronic diseases (Ghatak, 1931/1938, p. 7).

Homeopathy also explains the cause of internal problems. This also says when skin diseases are treated by external application of ointment and lotion, it is very dangerous. If external manifestations of psora, in the form of skin diseases, are treated externally, then they are redirected internally and responsible for diseases of internal organs. When a person is suffering from psora or syphilis or sycosis and then allopathic injection is given, it will direct the diseases internally and make them incurable (Ghatak, 1931/1938, pp. 7–9).

Now we can say that in homeopathy, the treatment of skin diseases by external application of ointment and lotion is strictly contraindicated. Similarly, injections also can never be given. Do you accept this concept?

A case of dysentery was described in homeopathy and it was said that this was treated by arsenic, in a homeopathic method, within 24 hours. An eight-year-old child was suffering from fever, thirst, and a watery stool with foul smell, 50–60 times a day. The child was given arsenic of 30th potency. Within 24 hours, the patient recovered. The credit was given to homeopathy (Ghatak, 1931/1938, pp. 14–15). But what was the truth? When a patient is suffering from fever, diarrhea, abdominal pain, diagnosis may be of shigellosis or bacillary dysentery. Other symptoms include nausea, vomiting, headache, myalgia, and respiratory symptoms. This disease is an acute, self-limited infection of the intestinal tract of humans, which is characterized by diarrhea, fever, and abdominal pain (Beaty, 1983, pp. 965–966).

There are various other causes of diarrhea. Diagnosis of specific etiological agents is done only by stool culture, where specific bacterial and viral agents can be seen by the microscope. Homeopathy does not accept external etiology of disease. Bacteria and viruses are not accepted by homeopathy as a cause of diseases; therefore, there is no question of specific diagnosis in homeopathy.

There are also other causes of diarrhea. Most of the types are self-limiting (Carpenter, 1983, pp. 885–889). Not only homeopathy but other

Chapter twenty two: Psora   77

useless pathies get unnecessary credit in these diarrhea like diseases, where diseases are actually self-limiting. In homeopathy, drugs are given in very dilute concentrations, and practically we can say that homeopathic drugs contain no drug.

Homeopathy also says that it is impossible to know about diseases. Homeopathy only involves patients and not diseases. It takes interest only in symptoms (Ghatak, 1931/1938, p. 15).

Homeopathy also says that the body of a person cannot be diseased without involving the thought process. Neither the body nor any organ can get disease until the psyche or thought process is not disturbed. Disease can spread only from the mind to the body. The body is actually an image of the mind. If the mind is pure, no disease can exist in the body (Ghatak, 1931/1938, pp. 20–21). It means that if a person has pure thought in his mind, he/she cannot suffer from any disease. It also indicates that all diseases such as cancer, organ enlargement, heart problems, thyroid disorders, diabetes, thyrotoxicosis, glomerulonephritis, and peptic ulcer are the result of disturbed psyche. According to homeopathy, disturbed psyche is responsible for damage in various organs and causes diseases.

Disease first starts in the mind, psyche, or desire, then it spreads in the body (Ghatak, 1931/1938, pp. 20–21). So when treatment is concerned, treat the psyche and desire of a patient. It is useless to treat disease in homeopathy, without treating psyche or thought. According to homeopathy, diseases actually start from inside to outside of the body. According to homeopathy, external factors like virus, bacteria, parasites, allergens, and environmental agents cannot produce any disease.

Homeopathy always says that tuberculosis, leprosy, typhoid, pneumonia, and other diseases are not caused by bacteria. They are caused by the wrong psyche and then spread from the mind to the body. The view of homeopathy is that bacteria and viruses have no capacity to produce diseases. First the disease is produced and then bacteria come and eat damaged portions of the organs (Ghatak, 1931/1938, p. 21).

Today, this is a false concept that bacteria and viruses are not responsible for any disease. Destruction of bacteria and viruses by sterilization, antibiotics, chemotherapeutic agents, and by vaccines improves the health status around the world. Spread of diseases, epidemics, and endemics are cured and checked by preventing spread of bacteria and viruses. Today we know that tropical diseases are caused by contaminated water. Epidemics occur after floods due to drinking of dirty water. As we also know that mosquitoes are responsible for malaria and filaria. If we accept homeopathy, then we shall have to agree with this concept that dirty water is not responsible for epidemics and mosquitoes do not cause malaria. Today we have proved evidence that mosquitoes cause malaria and bacteria cause diseases. This indicates that homeopathy is illogical, unscientific, and useless.

The given examples explain the pattern of treatment in homeopathy. Let's say that there are four patients. The first is suffering from bleeding in the stomach, the second is suffering from toothache with mild fever. The third patient is suffering from diarrhea, and the fourth patient is suffering from typhoid fever. If all these patients have common symptoms like mental agony, thirst, desire for heat, then the treatment of all four patients will be the same like arsenic. If all four patients are suffering from cholera with different mental symptoms, different desires, absence, or presence of mental peace, then the treatment of cholera will be different for different patients (Ghatak, 1931/1938, p. 22).

A typical concept of homeopathy is that first of all the mind is affected. Drugs and diseases both first influence the mind, then the body gets affected. According to homeopathy, if a drug or disease has no effect on the mind, it cannot influence the body.

Today we know that there are hundreds of diseases and drugs that do not influence the mind but directly affect the body. Hypertension, diabetes, malaria, asthma, tumors, kidney disease, and liver disease are a few examples of diseases, where the mind is not affected in the beginning.

Drugs acting on G.I.T., C.V.S., urogenital system, respiratory system, skin, and eyes do not influence the mind but directly influence organs and diseases are cured. All tropical diseases are usually cured by antibiotics and chemotherapeutic agents without influencing the mind. This proves that the concept of homeopathy is also wrong.

Homeopathy says that the external application of ointment or lotion in the skin diseases should be forbidden. Injections are also not indicated in this therapy. These procedures suppress the disease. The body ejects faults of the mind externally and makes the mind pure. By wrong treatments, external manifestations are suppressed and again redirected internally and responsible for damage in internal organs. Then it is wrongly understood that the disease has been cured (Ghatak, 1931/1938, p. 37).

References

Beaty, H. N. (1983). Shigellosis. In R. G. Petersdorf, R. D. Adams, E. Braunwald, K. J. Isselbacher, J. B. Martin, & J. D. Wilson (Eds.), *Harrison's principle of internal medicine* (10th ed., pp. 965–967). New Delhi, India: McGraw Hill.

Carpenter, C. C. J. (1983). Acute infectious diarrhoeal disease and bacterial food poisoning. In R. G. Petersdorf, R. D. Adams, E. Braunwald, K. J. Isselbacher, J. B. Martin, & J. D. Wilson (Eds.), *Harrison's principle of internal medicine* (10th ed., pp. 885–889). New Delhi, India: McGraw Hill.

Ghatak, N. (1938). *Cause and cure of chronic diseases* (4th ed.) (C. S. Pathak, Trans.). Kolkata, India: Dr. S.M. Bhattacharya. (Original work published in 1931).

chapter twenty three

Development of psora

Basic concept of homeopathy – twenty three

Jealousy, lack of love, disturbed peace, selfishness, unfairness, and unjustified attitude for others are the causative factors in the development of psora. Psora is the base of all diseases. Homeopathy divides all diseases into two groups: (a) new and (b) old. If new diseases are treated wrongly, they convert into old or chronic diseases.

Argument

Homeopathy divides all diseases into two groups: (a) new diseases and (b) old diseases. New diseases are those diseases that may be resolved automatically. Either the patient will die or the patient will be cured automatically. If the disease is strong, then the patient will die, but this disease will not remain in the body for a prolonged period. Old diseases are those diseases that cannot be cured automatically. Such diseases remain in the body in various forms for prolonged duration (Ghatak, 1931/1938, pp. 45–46).

Homeopathy also says that if new diseases are treated wrongly, they convert into older chronic disease. But what was the truth? A large number of viral and bacterial diseases are cured automatically. If immunity is less or virulence of causative organisms is great, then there will be complications and disease will not be cured automatically. Due to these complications, disease will remain in the body for prolonged duration. When these diseases are cured, then the homeopath says these diseases are new. When there are complications of disease, the homeopath says this is due to wrong treatment. It was the explanation given by homeopathy. At the time when homeopathy originated, pathogenesis of disease was not known. When homeopathy did not accept bacterial and viral etiology of diseases, then how they had studied pathogenesis of disease. Homeopathy says complications of new disease always develop due to wrong treatment. But it is not true. Few patients with acute diseases have complications due to a lack of immunity.

Chickenpox is a mild self-limiting disease. But this may be accompanied by severe complications. These include hemorrhage, pneumonia, encephalitis, and acute cerebellar ataxia (Park, 1997, pp. 117–118).

DOI: 10.1201/9781003228622-23

There are many other bacterial and viral diseases like chickenpox. Usually these infections are self-limiting. In a few cases, there are complications and it had been said wrongly that these were due to wrong treatment.

In those diseases where dehydration or blood loss is a problem, old allopathic treatment like shedding streams of blood and purgative complicates the diseases, e.g., in cholera. But in those diseases where blood loss or dehydration is not a problem, external application of mercurial ointment or cinchona bark or quinine can never convert diseases into chronic forms. Actually it was wrong observations by supporters of homeopathy. They understood complication of disease as complication of mismanagement.

Meanwhile Hahnemann also said. "A human healing art, for the restoration to the normal state of those innumerable abnormal conditions so often produced by the allopathic non healing art, there is not and cannot be" (Hahnemann, 1921/1993, pp. 164–165).

One absurd concept of homeopathy is psora. According to homeopathy, all diseases are modifications of psora. In the absence of psora, disease is not possible. Jealousy, lack of love, disturbed peace, selfishness, unfairness, and unjustified attitude for others are the causative factors for the development of psora. First mental stage of psora is developed. This mental itching of psora later appears on the surface in the form of physical itching. The presence of itching proves that there is psora in the body. During disease, the state of mind reflects in the body (Ghatak, 1931/1938, p. 58).

Hahnemann writes,

> The psora, the only real fundamental cause and producer of all the other numerous I may say innumerable forms of diseases which under the name of nervous debility, hysteria, hypochondriasis, mania, melancholia, madness, epilepsy, convulsion of all sorts, scoliosis, hypnosis, caries, cancer, neoplasm, gout, haemorrhoids, Jaundice, cyanosis, dropsy, amenorrhoea, haemorrhage from the stomach, nose, lung, bladder, asthma, ulceration of lungs, of impotence, and barrenness, of megrim, deafness, cataract, amaurosis, urinary calculus, paralysis, defect of senses and pains of thousands of kinds etc. (Hahnemann, 1921/1993, p. 168)

According to homeopathy and Hahnemann, all mentioned diseases are caused by only a single agent, psora. Today we know about etiology,

Chapter twenty three: Development of psora 81

pathology, diagnosis, investigation, and treatment of diseases. We find different causative factors in different diseases. It is absolutely wrong to say that only psora is the main cause of all diseases.

Hahnemann did not mention characteristic, morphology, and measurement of psora and even not provide evidence of its existence. It is also said that this

> Extremely ancient infecting agent has gradually passed in some hundreds of generations through many millions of human organisms and has thus attained an incredible development, renders it in some measure conceivable how it can now display such innumerable morbid forms in the great family of mankind. (Hahnemann, 1921/1993, p. 169)

Hahnemann discarded external etiological factors of diseases. According to homeopathy, external factors alone can never create a disease. According to homeopathy, a perfectly healthy man has no psora and then administration of HIV or rabies virus in his body will not develop AIDS or rabies in him. Because in the absence of psora, disease cannot be developed. Are supporters of homeopathy ready to have administered HIV virus in their body? If they are not ready, then they are actually making fraudulent claims because they apply principles of homeopathy on others but do not apply on themselves. According to homeopathy, they will not get AIDS by HIV virus.

References

Ghatak, N. (1938). *Cause and cure of chronic diseases* (4th ed.) (C. S. Pathak, Trans.).,Kolkata, India: Dr. S.M. Bhattacharya. (Original work published in 1931).

Hahnemann, S. (1993). *Organon of medicine* (6th ed.) (W. Boericke, Trans.). New Delhi, India: B. Jain Publishers. (Original work published in 1921).

Park, K. (1997). *Park's textbook of preventive and social medicine* (15th ed.). Jabalpur, India: Banarsidas Bhanot Publisher.

chapter twenty four

Skin diseases

Basic concept of homeopathy – twenty four

Homeopathy opposes external application of lotion or ointment in skin diseases. This pathy tells that skin diseases are not isolated problems; these are actually external manifestations of internal diseases. Local, surgical, and other treatments for skin disease are also not indicated in this therapy.

Argument

The important fact regarding homeopathy is that, diseases which are self-limiting, homeopaths claimed that they are treating such diseases by homeopathy, and the diseases that are not self-limiting, homeopaths say, become chronic due to wrong treatment of allopathy or no treatment.

As said by Hahnemann,

> The true natural chronic diseases are those that arise from a chronic miasm, which when left to themselves and unchecked by the employment of those remedies that are specific for them, always go on increasing and growing worse ... These excepting those produced by medical malpractice, are the most numerous and greatest scourges of the human race. (Hahnemann, 1921/1993, p 166)

Homeopathy also defines what the malpractice of allopathy is. Homeopathy opposes external application of lotion or ointment in skin diseases. According to homeopathy, skin diseases are external manifestations of psora. When these skin diseases are treated by external application of lotion and ointment, then these diseases are suppressed and directed internally and create severe internal diseases. According to this view, skin diseases are not isolated problems; these are actually a part or external manifestation of internal diseases (Ghatak, 1931/1938, pp. 79–80).

Conclusively we can say, those who are supporters of homeopathy should never use external applications of drugs in skin diseases. This means

DOI: 10.1201/9781003228622-24

84   *Homeopathy*

that either homeopathy is true or skin specialist is true. Both can never be correct. Both are opposite to each other.

Similarly, homeopathy also says that psora, gonorrhea, and syphilis are suppressed by wrong treatment and this suppression creates many complications in the human body.

Hahnemann also writes,

> It is not useful either in acute local diseases of recent origin or in local affections that have already existed a long time, to run in or apply external remedy, even though it be the specific and when used internally salutary by reason of its homeopathically, even although it should be at the same time administered internally. (Hahnemann, 1921/1993, p. 236)

"A product of psora which had hitherto remained latent in the interior, but has now burst forth of is on the point of developing into a palpable chronic disease" (Hahnemann, 1921/1993, p. 236). This concept of homeopathy tells that skin diseases are manifestations of psora and should not be suppressed.

"In chromic local maladies that are not obviously venereal the antipsoric internal treatment is more ever alone requisite" (Hahnemann, 1921/1993, p. 237). This statement suggests that non-venereal local diseases like boil, carbuncle, scabies, ringworm, local fungal infections, and bed sores are the external manifestations of psora and should not be treated locally. External treatment is prohibited in homeopathy and only internal treatment is advised.

It has also been said in homeopathy,

> If the remedy perfectly homeopathic to the disease had not yet been discovered at the time when the local symptoms were destroyed by a corrosive or desiccative external remedy or by the knife then the cases become much more difficult on account of the too indefinite (uncharacteristic and inconstant) appearance of the remaining symptoms for what might have contributed most to determine the selection of the most suitable remedy and its internal employment until the disease should have been completely annihilated, namely the external principal symptoms has been removed from other observation. (Hahnemann, 1921/1993, p. 239)

Chapter twenty four: Skin diseases   85

According to homeopathy, all local symptoms are part of some general or systemic diseases, and local problems should not be treated by external application of drugs or by surgery. According to homeopathy, the presence of disease in the body can be only diagnosed by external symptoms or visible external manifestations of disease. If external manifestations are removed by external application, then the homeopath cannot decide whether disease has been cured or remained in the body. By external application of drugs, diseases redirect from the external surface to interior of the body and create complications. That's why homeopathy opposes the external application of drug. "The mere topical employment of medicines that are powerful for cure when given internally to the local symptoms of chronic miasmatic diseases is for the same reason quite inadmissible" (Hahnemann, 1921/1993, p. 238).

Today we know that the above concept of homeopathy is not true. Many diseases are treated only by local treatment. Local abscess, cataract, conjunctivitis, glaucoma, deviated nasal septum, urethral stricture, phimosis, and localized carcinomatous growth are a few examples, where local treatment, surgical or medical is a must. These diseases cannot be cured by internal treatment. Homeopathy says that only external treatment, local morbidity or disease can never be treated. But at present, we know that only localized surgical or medicinal treatment can cure these above ailments.

References

Ghatak, N. (1938). *Cause and cure of chronic diseases* (4th ed.) (C. S. Pathak, Trans.). Kolkata, India: Dr S.M. Bhattacharya. (Original work published in 1931).

Hahnemann, S. (1993). *Organon of medicine* (6th ed.) (W. Boericke, Trans.). New Delhi, India: B. Jain Publishers. (Original work published in 1921).

chapter twenty five

Wart and localized treatment

Basic concept of homeopathy – twenty five

Warts are cured by the internal application of homeopathy medicines. Localized extirpation of carcinomatous growth should not be performed as it develops other internal complications.

Argument

Hahnemann writes,

> Persistence of local affections during its internal employment would have shown that the cure was not yet completed, but were it cured on its seat, this would be a convincing proof that the disease was completely eradicated of the desired recovery from the entire disease was fully accomplished, an estimable indispensable advantage to reach a perfect cure. (Hahnemann, 1921/1993, p. 240)

Homeopathy says, all local external diseases are part of generalized internal diseases. Its treatment presumes that by only external application of drugs, diseases cannot be cured. So, for total eradication of such diseases, drugs should be given orally. Homeopathy says that when external manifestations are removed after the internal application of a drug, the drug effect is established reliably.

To explore the concept of homeopathy, an example is given here. Warts are benign neoplasms of the skin, which are found in 7–20% of the population. They occur mainly on skin areas. Warts are caused by human papovaviruses, which may persist and spread within the same person for several years. Most studies indicate that one-third of warts are cured in six months and two-thirds of diseases are resolved spontaneously within a two-year period. As mentioned earlier, most warts usually disappear spontaneously without leaving any scars (Corey, 1983, pp. 1174–1180). In the affected persons, the diseases disappear spontaneously within 6–24 months. In cases of warts, if homeopathic drugs are given internally after presuming that warts are part of general disease, then this disease

DOI: 10.1201/9781003228622-25

will be cured spontaneously, but this is a false reputation claimed by homeopathy.

In the treatment of warts, homeopathic drugs are popularly accepted, although the reality is not known by persons that warts are usually cured spontaneously. Warts are strictly localized diseases and are cured spontaneously. Homeopathy falsely claims that warts are cured by the internal application of homeopathic drugs and makes the wrong concept that warts are a part of a general disease. In this way, the concept and credit of homeopathy depend on spontaneously curable diseases. As such homeopathy plays no role in therapeutics.

According to homeopathy, localized diseases are part of generalized diseases. Hahnemann further explains

> It is evident that man's vital force, when encumbered with a chronic disease which it is unable to overcome by its own powers, instinctively adopts the plan of developing a local malady on some external part ... It may thereby silence the internal disease which otherwise threatens to destroy the vital organs (and to deprive the patient of life) and that it may thereby, so to speak, transfer the internal disease to the vicarious local affection ... The local affection however is never anything else than a part of it increased all in one direction by the organic vital force and transferred to a less dangerous (external part) of the body in order to allay the internal ailment. (Hahnemann, 1921/1993, p. 240)

Hahnemann also did a wrong generalization of a few diseases such as syphilis. He said, "The chancre enlarges as long as the internal syphilis remains uncured, old ulcers on legs get worse as long as the internal Psora is uncured" (Hahnemann, 1921/1993, p. 242). In this way, he made generalizations of knowledge based on only a few diseases. In some cases, local affections may be part of general diseases, but it is not a universal truth. All local diseases are not part of general diseases. Homeopathy also opposes the external application of drugs.

Hahnemann writes,

> Physicians destroy the local symptoms by the topical application of external remedies, under the belief that he, thereby, cures the whole disease. Nature makes up for its loss by rousing the internal malady and the other symptoms that previously existed

Chapter twenty five: Wart and localized treatment   *89*

> in a latent state side by side with the local affec-
> tion that is to say though incorrectly that the local
> affection has been driven back into system or upon
> the nerves by the external remedies. (Hahnemann,
> 1921/1993, p. 242)

He also writes, "Burning away the chancre by caustics and destroying
the condylomata on their seat by knife, the ligature or the actual cautery,
this pernicious external mode of treatment ... is one of the most criminal
procedures the medical world can be guilty of" (Hahnemann, 1921/1993,
p. 242).

If homeopathy is true, then the external treatment of localized affection should not be performed – neither by surgery nor by injections or
drugs. If this concept of homeopathy is true, then skin specialists should
not prescribe any local remedy, and orthopedicians should not use any
local applications for nontraumatic localized diseases. It also says, localized carcinomatous growth should not be removed by surgery.

Why does homeopathy oppose localized treatment? Because home-
opathy concludes that localized treatment cannot cure localized diseases.
It always aggravates the disease and deteriorates the condition of patients.
Hahnemann also opposes local treatment by surgery.

Hahnemann writes,

> I cannot advise for instance the local extirpation of
> the so called cancer of the lips and face ... the basic
> malady is, thereby, not diminished in slightest, the
> preserving vital force is, therefore, necessitated to
> transfer the field of operation of the great internal
> malady to some more important part (as it does in
> every case of metastasis) and the consequence is
> blindness, deafness, insanity, suffocative asthma ...
> The result is the same without previous cure of
> the inner miasm when cancer of the face or breast
> is removed by the knife alone and when encysted
> tumors are enucleated. Something worse ensues
> or at any rate death is hastened. (Hahnemann,
> 1921/1993, p. 244)

Today we know that the best and only treatment of carcinomatous
growth is surgery. The previous conclusion of Hahnemann was wrong.
Hahnemann did not know the pathogenesis of the spread of cancer. In
most of the cancer cases, metastasis occurs. Cancer usually spreads via
lymph, blood into lung, liver, brain, bone, and other parts of the body.

If carcinomatous growth is removed in an early stage, it does not spread; and if there is delay in the removal of growth, it spreads in the body. Hahnemann wrongly assumed that it was the surgical removal of cancer that was responsible for the spread of cancer in the body and this was not the real treatment because, even after surgical treatment, patients suffered from metastatic growth. Due to lack of knowledge, Hahnemann got wrong impressions and presented the wrong pathy to the world.

Hahnemann also concluded wrongly that the external removal of carcinomatous growth produces other internal diseases. Actually, the fact is that if there is any carcinomatous growth of the advanced stage, there will be metastasis. Even after the removal of carcinomatous growth by surgery, these metastases that are already present in different parts of the body produce different signs and symptoms according to the organ involved. The pattern of metastatic spread is different in various cancers. If a part of cancer reaches the brain, neurological signs and symptoms will be the outcome. If metastatic growth reaches the lung, respiratory problems will be the result. In this way, different types of signs and symptoms will be produced according to the organ involved. Hahnemann said by mistake that these different types of signs and symptoms are the result of different types of internal diseases produced due to the removal of carcinomatous growth by surgery. Here Hahnemann was absolutely wrong to deliver the wrong message to the world.

References

Corey, L. (1983). Warts and molluscum contagiosum. In R. G. Petersdorf, R. D. Adams, E. Braunwald, K. J. Isselbacher, J. B. Martin, & J. D. Wilson (Eds.), *Harrison's principle of internal medicine* (10th ed., pp. 1174–1180). New Delhi, India: McGraw Hill.

Hahnemann, S. (1993). *Organon of medicine* (6th ed.) (W. Boericke, Trans.). New Delhi, India: B. Jain Publishers. (Original work published in 1921).

chapter twenty six

Psychiatric symptoms

Basic concept of homeopathy – twenty six

Rapid increases of the psychiatric symptoms are related to improvement in corporal symptoms. Hahnemann prescribed aconite, belladonna, hyoscyamus, and mercury in highly potentized minute homeopathic doses.

Argument

Hahnemann indicates regarding allopathic treatment of psychiatric patients. In allopathy, psychiatric patients are managed by harsh and cruel behavior. Physical tortures are given to them and they behave like criminals (Hahnemann, 1921/1996, p. 198).

Hahnemann rightly criticized the treatment of old allopathy. The earliest treatment of mental disorder was exorcism that included prayer, incantation, noise making, flogging, torture, starving, and other more severe measures. There were also patients who were beheaded or strangled before being burned, burned alive, and some were mutilated before being burned (Coleman, 1976, pp. 25–36).

But today, these methods are not used in the treatment of psychiatric patients. In modern medical science, which is also called modern allopathy, for the treatment of psychiatric patients, drugs, psychotherapy, and sociotherapy are used. These methods are human methods. A large percentage of psychiatric patients can be cured completely and they are able to live normal lives.

Now again we can say, Hahnemann opposed old allopathy. At the time of Hahnemann, there was no existence of modern and developed medical science. So this statement that Hahnemann opposed modern medical science is absolutely wrong.

Hahnemann writes,

> Almost all the so-called mental and emotional diseases are nothing more than corporeal diseases in which the symptoms of derangement of the mind and disposition peculiar to each of them is increased whilst the corporeal symptoms decline …
> The cases are not rare in which a so-called corporeal

> that threatens to be fatal a suppuration of lung or the deterioration of some other important viscous or some other disease of acute character ... becomes transformed into insanity, into a kind or melancholia or into mania by a rapid increase of the psychiatric symptoms that were previously present whereupon the corporeal symptoms lose all their danger, these latter improve almost to perfect health. (Hahnemann, 1921/1993, pp. 215–216)

These observations of Hahnemann were wrong. It does not mean that Hahnemann was not intelligent. He was definitely very intelligent, but due to the lack of necessary information and poor available knowledge, he was unable to reach the right conclusion.

At present, we know that all mental and emotional diseases are not the result of corporeal diseases. Some psychiatric symptoms are the result of organic diseases. One example is delirium. It is characterized by clouding of consciousness, perceptual disturbance, incoherent speech, impairment of memory and orientation, variation in clinical features, and most importantly, a specific organic factor. Mortality is due to the nature of disease that causes delirium. Progression to irreversible organic brain damage is also observed, where the etiology cannot be treated effectively (Wells, 1985).

When psychiatric symptoms increase, the intensity of corporeal disease does not decline in cases of delirium. If organic diseases, responsible for delirium, are not treated effectively, then it increases the chances of death. This conclusion is against the "Organon of Medicine" which says that when psychiatric symptoms increase, corporeal symptoms lose all their danger. For the treatment of delirium Hahnemann prescribed, "aconite, belladonna hyoscyamus, mercury, stramonium in highly potentized, minute homeopathic doses" (Hahnemann, 1921/1993, p. 253). These drugs prescribed for the treatment of delirium, when given in high doses, produce delirium with other toxic signs and symptoms. Aconite produces "sometimes delirium or convulsion, insensibility and coma" (Modi, 1975, p. 742).

> By stramonium, hypocrite and belladonna, in high doses, patient becomes restless, markedly excited and delirious. Delirium is of particular character. He is silent or mutters indistinct inaudible words but usually he is noisy, tries to run away from his bed, tries to pull imaginary threads from the tips of his fingers and is subject to dreadful hallucinations of sight and hearing. (Modi, 1975, p. 697)

Chapter twenty six: Psychiatric symptoms   93

During mercury poisoning "neuropsychiablic symptoms also occur" (Klaassen, 1980, p. 1624). These all drugs produce delirium and other psychiatric symptoms when given in toxic doses, but these drugs cannot cure delirium. When drugs are given in homeopathic doses, in high dilutions, they have no effect on the human body, neither therapeutic nor toxic.

Homeopathic dose means that drug is given in high dilution. But Hahnemann got some positive results from these drugs in delirium.

There are various causes of delirium. Bacterial, viral infections, and toxic doses of various drugs also cause delirium. Many infections like typhoid and viral infections are self-limiting. Toxic substances, responsible for delirium, gradually metabolize in the body and delirium subsides spontaneously, if there is no irreversible damage in the brain. Systemic infections like fever also cause delirium. As infections and fever are cured, it also gets cured. In this way, delirium may resolve automatically without any treatment. Under such conditions homeopathy gets a pseudo reputation as a treating agent.

Facts about delirium should be known to all. "It is not too unusual for delirium to come and go without a specific cause being identified" (Wells, 1985, p. 848). Actually,

> Acute brain disorders are caused by diffuse impairment of brain function. Such impairment may result from a variety of conditions including high fevers, nutritional deficiency and drug intoxication. Symptoms range from mild mood changes to acute delirium. The prognosis in acute brain disorder is good. Such conditions usually clear up over a short period of time. (Coleman, 1976, p. 460)

Actually the fact is that if a patient is cured by homeopathy, then it is said, it is a homeopathic drug that is responsible for cure, irrespective of spontaneous cure of disease. If disease is not cured by homeopathic drugs, then it is said that allopathic drugs or some other treatments have spoiled the case.

References

Coleman, J. (1976). *Abnormal psychology and modern life*. Bombay, India: Taraporewala and Sons.

Hahnemann, S. (1993). *Organon of medicine* (6th ed.) (W. Boericke, Trans.). New Delhi, India: B. Jain Publishers. (Original work published in 1921).

Hahnemann, S. (1996). *Organon of medicine* (6th ed.) (P. Devi, Trans.). New Delhi, India: B. Jain Publishers. (Original work published in 1921).

Klaassen, C. D. (1980). Heavy metals and heavy metals antagonists. In A. G. Gilman, L. Goodman, & A. Gilman (Eds.), *Goodman and Gilman's pharmacological basis of therapeutics* (6th ed., pp. 1615–1637). New York, NY: Macmillan.

Modi, N. J. (1975). *Textbook of medical jurisprudence and toxicology* (9th ed.). Bombay, India: N.M. Tripathi, Publisher

Wells, C. E. (1985). Organic syndromes: Delirium. In H. I. Kaplan, & B. J. Sadock (Eds.), *Comprehensive textbook of psychiatry* (4th ed., pp. 838–851). Baltimore, MD: Williams and Wilkins.

chapter twenty seven

Dynamization

Basic concept of homeopathy – twenty seven

According to homeopathy, dilution and trituration increase the potency of a drug. The material part of the medicine is lessened with each degree of dynamization of 50,000 times and yet incredibly increased in power. The 30th thus progressively prepared would give a fraction almost impossible to be expressed in number but highly potent in power.

Argument

Dynamization means to give power or energy to inert material and potentiation means to increase its strength.

> Homeopathic system of medicine develops … a process peculiar to it … Whereby only they become immeasurably and penetratingly efficacious, even those that in the crude state give no evidence of the slightest medicinal power on the human body … This is effected by mechanical action upon their smallest particles by means of rubbing and shaking and through addition of an indifferent substance, dry and fluid are separated from each other. This process is called dynamizing, potentiating (development of medicinal power). (Hahnemann, 1921/2017, pp. 219–220)

Hahnemann further says, by only dilution, medicinal power cannot be developed. Hidden medicinal power is brought forth by rubbing, shaking, and trituration, and in this way, the well-being of animal life can be improved. He mentioned an example of magnetism, in his support, where an iron bar after rubbing with a magnet develops power of magnetism (Hahnemann, 1921/2017, pp. 220–221).

Now it is the method of preparing homeopathic medicine. It is said that by this method, crude medicinal substances develop their curative power to the utmost, which is as follows. One grain of the powdered drug is triturated with 100 grains of sugar of milk. The powder thus prepared

DOI: 10.1201/9781003228622-27

95

96   *Homeopathy*

is put in a vial well-corked, protected from direct sunlight to which the designation of the first product marked 1/100 is given. Now 1 grain of the powdered 1/100 is mixed and triturated with 100 grains of powdered sugar and labeled 1/10,000 (2c potency) and again 1 grain of this powder is taken, mixed, and triturated with 100 grains of sugar of milk and labeled 1/1,000,000 (3c potency). Now again 1 grain of this powder is dissolved in 500 drops of a mixture of one part (100 drops) of alcohol and four parts of distilled water (400 drops) of which one drop is put in a vial. This is LM/0 potency. To this are added 100 drops of pure alcohol and 100 strong succussions are given. This is the medicine of the first degree of dynamization, LM/1. After spreading and drying on a blotting paper, take one globule and mix with 100 drops of good alcohol and dynamize in the same way with 100 powerful succussions. Repeat this process 30 times and prepare a drug of LM 30 potency (Hahnemann, 1921/2017, pp. 222–223).

Regarding such dilution, Hahnemann writes,

> I have found after many laborious experiments and counter experiments, to be the most powerful and at the same time mildest in action, i.e. as the most perfected, the material part of the medicine is lessened with each degree of dynamization 50000 times and yet incredibly increased in power ... The thirtieth thus progressively prepared would give a fraction almost impossible to be expressed in numbers. (Hahnemann, 1921/2017, pp. 224–225)

Homeopathic drugs contain such dilutions that practically contain no drug at all. Homeopathic drugs have no curative and therapeutic power. In other words, these drugs have no effect on the body. Hahnemann says by succussion, medicinal power of a drug is increased. With knowledge of physics, we know by succussion, only mechanical energy is produced, which is responsible for a slight increase in temperature and nothing else.

> In homeopathy, dilutions are based on a 1:10 ratio represented by the Roman numeral X or D, and centesimal based on a 1:100 ratio by the Roman letter C. Hence a 1 X homeopathic dosage is 10-fold dilution, 2X is a 100-fold dilution, 3X is a 1000-fold dilution, etc. The 1C represents a 100-fold dilution, 2C is a 10,000- fold dilution and 3C is a 1,000,000-fold dilution etc. Most homeopathic remedies range from 6X (one part in a million) to 30 X (one part in 10^{30}). (Marderosian et al., 2000, p. 1771)

Chapter twenty seven: Dynamization 97

> Centesimal scale involves a serial dilution 1/100 whereas decimal involves a serial trituration 1/10: 1c potency equal to 1/100 dilution, 1x potency equal to 1/10 dilution, 6x potency equal to $1/10^6$ dilution, 6c potency equal to $1/10^{12}$ dilution, 12x potency equal to $1/10^{12}$, 30 c potency equal to $1/10^{60}$, 200 c dilution equal to $1/10^{400}$, 1000 c (1M) potency equal to $1/10^{2000}$, 10000 c (10 M) equal to $1/10^{20000}$ dilution. (Banerjee, 1999, p. 48)

In such dilutions, there is actually no drug molecule. When there is no drug molecule, how can we expect an effect on the body?

> According to the laws of chemistry, there is a point at which a substance can be diluted so that no more remains. The limit is referred to as Avogadro's number, which closely corresponds to the homeopathic dosage of 24 X (one part in 10^{24}). Even Hahnemann recognized that in all likelihood, extreme dilutions would not contain a single molecule of the original material. (Marderosian et al., 2000, p. 1771)

References

Banerjee, D. D. (1999). *A textbook of homeopathic pharmacy*. New Delhi, India: B. Jain Publishers.

Hahnemann, S. (2017). *Organon of medicine* (6th ed.) (W. Boericke, Trans.). New Delhi, India: B. Jain Publishers. (Original work published in 1921).

Marderosian, A. H. D., Krantz, A. M., & Riedlinger, J. E. (2000). Complementary & alternative medical health care. In A. R. Gennaro (Ed.), *Remington: The science and practice of pharmacy* (20th ed., Vol. 2, pp. 1762–1779). Philadelphia, PA: Lippincott Williams and Wilkins.

chapter twenty eight

Fever, injection, and vaccination

Basic concept of homeopathy – twenty eight

Homeopathy opposes the treatment of fever. Tuberculosis and similar diseases are developed when fever is treated. This pathy says that only the presence of symptoms indicates the disease. If investigations indicate the disease but there are no symptoms, then homeopathy would not accept the disease. During treatment the mind should be cured first, and then the body is cured. Homeopaths criticized injections and vaccination and also report that these procedures are very dangerous.

Argument

Homeopathy opposes the treatment of fever. Homeopathy says that the size of the liver and spleen is increased when fever is treated. Similarly, TB and other similar diseases also develop when fever is treated (Ghatak, 1931/1938, pp. 81–82). Today we know that temperature above 102°F is dangerous to the body. Hyperpyrexia is also responsible for death. But homeopathy says that fever should not be treated because tuberculosis-like diseases are originated due to the treatment of fever. This is the finding of homeopathy.

Homeopathy says that if external symptoms of disease are improved but the patient is not feeling well and not calm and quiet, then the patient is not improving (Ghatak, 1931/1938). In this case, treatment is not accurate. This pathy says that if external symptoms (like fever, pain, frequency of stool, cough, dyspnea) are increased in severity and the patient feels better, then it indicates the patient is improving (Ghatak, 1931/1938). The mechanism of the above action is explained as follows. First, drug acts inside the body and patients feel better, and then the drug acts outside. The action of the drug starts from inside to outside, that's why first the patient feels good, then symptoms are removed. Persons having little knowledge of medical science know well that first external symptoms are improved, then only patients feel better. For example, if a patient is suffering from a fever of 105°F, first we have to reduce his temperature, then only the patient will feel better. But it is not possible that the first patient feels better then only the temperature will be reduced. Similarly, if a patient is suffering from severe pain, without removing pain the patient cannot feel good.

DOI: 10.1201/9781003228622-28

100   *Homeopathy*

Improvements in external symptoms like pain, fever, and swelling are definite signs of cure but homeopathy denies this concept. How a patient can improve or feel well when he is suffering from severe pain, high-grade temperature, or deteriorating symptomatology.

Homeopaths criticized vaccination and injections. According to these experts, vaccination and injections create various complications and also report that these procedures are very dangerous (Ghatak, 1931/1938, p. 223). But we know that injections of various medicines are lifesaving in emergencies. Besides, many drugs are administered only by injections. Vaccinations are highly beneficial in preventing many infectious diseases. In vaccinations, vaccines are administered, which prevent the development of disease. Vaccine is an immunobiological substance, designed to produce specific protection against a given disease. It stimulates the production of protective antibodies of other immune mechanisms. Smallpox, rabies, cholera, diphtheria, TB, pertussis, tetanus, influenza, yellow fever, mumps, polio, measles, rubella, and hepatitis-B vaccines are used in the prevention of respective diseases. In May 1974, the WHO officially launched an immunization program to protect all children of the world against six vaccine-preventable diseases, diphtheria, whooping cough, tetanus, polio, tuberculosis, and measles by 2000.

One effective way of controlling the infection is to strengthen the host defenses. This may be accomplished by active immunization that is one of the most effective weapons of modern medicine. There are many infectious diseases and their control is solely based on active immunization, e.g., polio, tetanus, diphtheria, and measles. Immunization is a successful means of protecting the greatest number of people (Park, 1997, pp. 91–100).

Today if an expert or a pathy opposes vaccinations and says vaccination and immunization are harmful, then we can say that these persons do not know anything about medical science and these pathies are useless.

References

Ghatak, N. (1938). *Cause and cure of chronic diseases* (4th ed.) (C. S. Pathak, Trans.). Kolkata, India: Dr. S.M. Bhattacharya. (Original work published in 1931).

Park, K. (1997). *Park's textbook of preventive and social medicine* (15th ed.). Jabalpur, India: Banarsidas Bhanot Publisher.

chapter twenty nine

Suffering with two dissimilar diseases

Basic concept of homeopathy – twenty nine

If two dissimilar diseases meet together in the human being of equal strength or if the older one is the stronger, the new disease will be repelled by the old one from the body and not allowed to affect it or strong disease suppresses another weak disease. When strong disease is cured, weak disease reappears.

Argument

Hahnemann made some observations, and on the basis of these observations, Hahnemann developed homeopathy. At the time of Hahnemann, medical science was not developed. Etiology, pathogenesis, specific diagnosis, and investigations were not well known. Hahnemann himself did not believe in diagnosis, investigations, pathogenesis, and exogenous etiological agents. Detailed analysis of concepts provided by Hahnemann is a must to understand; what is homeopathy and why is it wrong?

Hahnemann made this conclusion. "If the two dissimilar diseases meeting together in the human being be of equal strength or still more if the older one be the stronger, the new disease will be repelled by the old one from the body and not allowed to affect it" (Hahnemann, 1921/1993, p. 117). This conclusion of Hahnemann was also based on the following observations (Hahnemann, 1921/1993, pp. 117–132).

1. A patient suffering from a severe chronic disease will not be infected by a moderate autumnal dysentery or other epidemic diseases.
2. Those sufferings from pulmonary tuberculosis are not liable to be attacked by an epidemic fever of a not very violent character.
3. Pulmonary phthisis remained stationary when the patient was attacked by a violent typhus.
4. In an epidemic, measles attacked many individuals on the fourth and fifth days after the inoculation of smallpox and prevented the development of smallpox.

DOI: 10.1201/9781003228622-29

5. The mumps immediately disappears when the cowpox inoculation has taken effect.
6. Smallpox coming on after vaccination at once removed entirely the cowpox homeopathically.
7. The fever accompanying cowpox cured homeopathically intermittent fever in two individuals.
8. In some, two fevers cannot coexist in the same body.
9. In an epidemic where measles and whooping cough prevailed, many children who took measles remained free from whooping cough, etc. Hahnemann also said that many diseases have been homeopathically cured by other diseases presenting similar symptoms.

Today we can say with the help of advanced medical science, by the symptoms only, a disease cannot be diagnosed with confirmation. For diagnosis of infective diseases, viral and bacterial isolation and its confirmation microscopically or by a serological test is a must. Hahnemann has made this mistake and concluded wrong interpretations after wrong diagnosis or observing one or two or a few cases.

Immunity plays a very important role in the development of a disease. Hahnemann did not know about immunity and antigen-antibody reaction; that's why he did not understand the mechanism of the above observations. In the development of a disease, resistance of the host is very important. Resistance means the ability to localize and destroy microorganism. This capacity is dependent upon the presence of specific antibody that synthesizes in response to a specific antigenic stimulus. Variations in host resistance are the result of the host's ability to form antibodies. Malnutrition (especially protein deficiency), toxic depression due to bacterial toxins, and hormonal imbalance can greatly depress synthesis of antibodies. Anything that reduces the number of leukocytes also reduces resistance.

Very young and very old persons are much more susceptible to bacterial disease. New-born infant has little capacity for producing antibodies until he is several months of age.

> Presence of other diseases may greatly reduce resistance to bacterial infection. Diabetic patients are predisposed to infections of skin and genito-urinary tract. Influenza, measles and other viral infections of the lung markedly predispose to secondary bacterial infection. Silicosis is associated with a striking increase in susceptibility to tuberculosis. Malnutrition, exhaustion, shock, exposure to cold, chronic alcoholism, psychic disturbances etc. may also seriously interfere with the individual resistance to bacterial disease. (Hoppes, 1971, p. 275)

Chapter twenty nine: *Suffering with two dissimilar diseases* 103

"Prior contact with an organism or its product whether by active infection or by artificial immunization increases resistance to some infections such as measles, diphtheria and pertussis by stimulating antibody production" (Petersdorf, 1983, p. 841). We also know today that immunity creates a resistant state but some forms of immune reaction can produce severe and occasionally fatal results; it is known as hypersensitivity reaction. It is actually an inappropriate response to an antigenic stimulus, which may be a self-molecule or a drug or microbial product. Microbial product means product from bacteria, virus, protozoa or other microorganisms. Examples are salmonella infection, tubercular infection, leprosy, and streptococcal infection. Clinical manifestations depend upon where the antigen-antibody complexes form or lodge. In hypersensitivity reaction, eczema, skin rashes, pyrexia, and arthralgia may be developed. These events occur in drug ingestion, bacterial and viral infection (Greenwood et al., 1997, pp. 142–145).

"Immunity also plays a protective role in polio and a number of other viral infections. Immunity to many viral infections is life long" (Greenwood et al., 1997, p. 149). "It is also known that infections with influenza, rubella, measles and other viruses predisposes to bacterial and other infection" (Greenwood et al., 1997, p. 151). "Susceptibility to infection is generally greater in being young and old because of a weaker immune response. However, the immunopathology tends to be less severe" (Greenwood et al., 1997, p. 152). "Natural infection with a virus is an extremely effective means of giving life long immunity from the disease. In most cases where there is one virus type, it means that second attacks are extremely rare" (Greenwood et al., 1997, p. 153). "Because of the intimate relationship of viruses to the metabolism of their host cells, immunity may be raised or lowered by nutritional changes, endocrine disturbances, heat, cold, shock, radiation and other factors that stimulate or inhibit the activity of intracellular enzymes" (Pinkerton, 1971, p. 378).

These facts of antigen-antibody reaction in viral and bacterial infection were missed by Hahnemann. If immunity is strong, then some diseases may be totally asymptomatic, e.g., "Rubella is a mild self limiting viral disease and there is evidence that the disease may be entirely asymptomatic and detectable only by leukopenia and lymph node enlargement" (Pinkerton, 1971, p. 396). This shows that disease may exist in the body without any symptoms. In such conditions, Hahnemann may have thought about the absence of disease and made wrong conclusions but in fact there was disease.

Viral infections usually have characteristically specific skin lesions. In some viral infections, skin lesions are the only manifestations, e.g., chicken pox. "In the great majority of cases the cutaneous eruption is the only lesion seen" (Pinkerton, 1971, p. 394), as seen in measles.

"There are erythematous cutaneous eruptions of a characteristic appearance" (Pinkerton, 1971, p. 395). "Herpes zoster, commonly known as shingles, is characterized by the formation of an erythematous and vesicular eruption along the course of sensory nerves" (Pinkerton, 1971, p. 394). Similarly, smallpox and chickenpox have characteristic skin lesions. It is also known that "Antigen antibody reactions are important in causing cutaneous eruption e.g., note the absence of rashes in measles when antibodies do not form" (Pinkerton, 1971, p. 393). That's why we can say when antigen-antibody reaction is weak, then skin manifestations will be less and organs where antigen-antibody complex causes damage will also be less. In such conditions, diagnosis of disease is difficult due to the absence of characteristically specific skin lesions and less morbidity due to diminished antigen-antibody reaction or less hypersensitivity reaction.

Hahnemann did not know about the complexity of immunity and antigen-antibody reaction. Definitely, he made mistakes regarding the presence and absence of disease and got the wrong conclusion. Hahnemann observed that two dissimilar diseases cannot exist together. This observation was based on the absence of one disease. If cutaneous lesions are absent and morbidity is less, then one may think of the absence of disease because, at the time of Hahnemann, these were the only criteria for the presence or absence of disease in the body but absent cutaneous lesions and diminished morbidity gave wrong impression that disease is absent. Definitely, this was the mistake done by Hahnemann and he thought wrongly that one disease cures a similar disease but in fact one disease diminishes immunity, which makes antigen-antibody reaction less strong. This gives the false impression that disease is absent.

This explanation can be easily understood with the help of AIDS and tuberculosis patients.

> Tuberculin is a test material or antigen derived from tubercular bacteria when injected intradermally in the forearm, a positive reaction consisting of erythema and induration is accepted as evidence of past or present infection by mycobacterium tuberculosis. It is actually an antigen antibody reaction. If cellular immunity is poor then by negative tuberculin test tuberculosis cannot be excluded. The dermal hypersensitivity to tuberculin can also be lost in various states of immune suppression e.g. malignancy, Hodgkin's disease (Park, 1997, p. 142).

AIDS, the acquired immunodeficiency syndrome, is a fatal illness caused by a retrovirus known as the human immunodeficiency virus that destroys the body's immune system. Then the patient becomes vulnerable to various dangerous infections, neurological disorders, and

Chapter twenty nine: Suffering with two dissimilar diseases 105

malignancies. HIV-infected patients (that is, human immunodeficiency virus infection or HIV infection that causes AIDS),

> with tuberculosis have a higher frequency of false negative tuberculin skin test. HIV positive people with pulmonary tuberculosis may have a higher frequency of negative sputum smears. In people with HIV, who do not have a fully functioning immune system, there is less tissue destruction and hence less lung cavitation. Cavities usually develop because of the immune response to the tubercular bacilli. (Park, 1997, p. 150)

Decreased immunity is responsible for less damage in only those organs where the antigen-antibody complex is responsible for the destruction of tissue. It does not mean that there are no symptoms or there is no disease or disease will remain symptomless. Microorganisms also produce detrimental effects in the body by various other methods like toxins, interference in cellular metabolism, and septicemia. Decreased immunity by the first infection interfered in skin manifestations, and in some cases, it may decrease symptomatology that confused Hahnemann who then made the wrong interpretation.

I am again explaining one example of how Hahnemann made a wrong conclusion. Due to a lack of knowledge, Hahnemann writes,

> Smallpox coming on after vaccination as its great similarity at once removed entirely the cow pox homeopathically and does not permit it to come to maturity but on the other hand the cow pox when near maturity does. On account of its great similarity homeopathically diminish very much the supervening smallpox and make it much milder. (Hahnemann, 1921/1993, p. 130)

Hahnemann concluded that cowpox and smallpox both prevent the development of one other. Both diseases have similar symptomatology. So Hahnemann said that one disease homeopathically cured other diseases. Hahnemann gave emphasis on similar symptomatology, but what was the truth? It was not the similarity in symptomatology of cowpox and smallpox, which cured each other. It was the immunological and serological similarity of both types of viruses. Smallpox is due to variola virus. Cowpox is also a viral disease. By knowledge of pathology, we know, "Cowpox virus resembles that of smallpox morphologically and immunologically and the

106   Homeopathy

histological changes in the skin at the site of vaccination are essentially
identical with those of smallpox" (Pinkerton, 1971, p. 394).

Cowpox virus and smallpox virus both are similar immunologically;
this means both have similar antigenic structures. They make common
antibodies. Antibodies developed after cowpox inoculation prevent the
development of smallpox and vice versa. It is not the similarity in symptomatology but the similarity in (immunological) an antigenic structure
that prevents other diseases by the formation of common antibodies.
Cowpox virus develops antibodies that also kill smallpox virus. And
smallpox viruses develop antibodies that also kill cowpox viruses. This is
the actual mechanism.

Empirical observation of benefit in a few cases and actual therapeutic
benefit are two different aspects, as made clear by the following paragraph.
"In the past vaccinia virus has also been occasionally used for the treatment of disease such as recurrent herpes simplex infection or warts. There
is no evidence of therapeutic efficacy in these situations and the use of the
virus for these purposes is strictly contraindicated" (Corey, 1983, p. 1120).

Hahnemann says that two dissimilar diseases cannot exist in the
body together and he himself mentioned such examples that are against
the homeopathic concept. "Smallpox and measles, both these dissimilar
diseases were present at the same time. There was also a case where cowpox ran its regular course along with measles and along with purpura"
(Hahnemann, 1921/1993, p. 125). There are many examples of dissimilar
diseases that exist together. Diabetes patients also suffer from malaria,
hypertension, cardiac problems, and other diseases. Hypertensive patients
also suffer from infective disease or other nontropical diseases like cancer, renal, and cardiac diseases. According to homeopathy, if a person is
suffering from a chronic disease, then during this period, he cannot suffer
from any other diseases having dissimilar symptomatology. What homeopathy says is absolutely wrong.

By the knowledge of interferon, we can analyze various observations
of Hahnemann. Hahnemann did not know about interferon; that's why he
made many wrong conclusions. Interferons are species specific to cellular
glycoprotein, produced naturally by virus-infected cells, and have antiviral protective action. They are capable of interfering with a wide variety of viruses. They can therefore be considered potent broad-spectrum
antiviral compounds (Satoskar & Bhandarkar, 1999, pp. 773–774). "Certain
agents like the live attenuated measles virus, bacterial endotoxins, other
microbial extracts, polysaccharides can stimulate the production of endog-
enous interferon" (Satoskar & Bhandarkar, 1999, p. 774).

> The enhanced production of the antiviral proteins
> called interferons is one of the body's earliest

Chapter twenty nine: Suffering with two dissimilar diseases 107

responses to a viral infection. It is thought that the interferons help contain viral infections until the immune system can be fully activated. All cells appear to have the capacity to produce these substances after exposure to appropriate stimulus, virus, a protozoan parasite, lipo polysaccharides or an antibiotic such as kanamycin is all that is needed to increase a cell's rate of interferon synthesis. It is known that interferon can prevent viruses from reproducing. The interferons in addition to being used to treat viral infections are being extensively investigated for use in AIDS and Cancer therapy. (Dyke, 1997. pp. 611–612)

"Interferons may ameliorate viral infections by exerting direct antiviral effect and/or by modifying the immune response to infection" (Hayden, 1996, p. 1211). From the above studies, it is clear that viral and protozoal infections create interferon in host. That interferon prevents or suspends the next consequent viral infection by antiviral action. This fact was not known to Hahnemann that one infection prevents the next infection by producing interferon. When Hahnemann observed in viral diseases that one infection prevents the second infection of similar symptomatology, he made the wrong concept that one disease is cured by a disease of similar symptomatology. He applied this observation in all diseases, which was wrong.

Protozoal infection also develops interferon that can prevent further viral infection. Interferon is also synthesized by various other stimulatory agents. This is sufficient to tell that the conclusion of Hahnemann was not accurate because one viral infection may prevent the development of another viral or bacterial infection irrespective of similarity or dissimilarity in symptomatology.

References

Corey, L. (1983). Warts and molluscum contagiosum. In R. G. Petersdorf, R. D. Adams, E. Braunwald, K. J. Isselbacher, J. B. Martin, & J. D. Wilson (Eds.), *Harrison's principle of internal medicine* (10th ed., pp. 1174–1180). New Delhi, India: McGraw Hill.

Dyke, K. V. (1997). Antiviral drugs. In C. R. Craig, & R. E. Stitzel (Eds.), *Modern pharmacology with clinical applications* (5th ed., pp. 605–612). New York, NY: Little Brown and Company.

Greenwood, D., Slack, R., & Peutherer, J. (Eds.) (1997). *Medical microbiology* (14th ed) eds.). New York, NY: Churchill Livingstone.

Hahnemann, S. (1993). *Organon of medicine* (6th ed.) (W. Boericke, Trans.). New Delhi, India: B. Jain Publishers. (Original work published in 1921).

Hayden, F. G. (1996). Antiviral agents. In J. G. Hardman, L. E. Limbird, P. B. Molinoff, R. W. Ruddon, & A. G. Gilman (Eds.), *Goodman and Gilman's pharmacological basis of therapeutics* (6th ed., pp. 1191–1223). NewYork, NY: McGraw-Hill.

Hoppes, H. C. (1971). Bacterial diseases. In W.A.D. Anderson (Ed.), *Pathology* (6th ed., Vol. 1, pp. 270–372). St. Louis, MO: C.V. Mosby Company.

Park, K. (1997). *Park's textbook of preventive and social medicine* (15th ed.). Jabalpur, India: Banarsidas Bhanot Publisher.

Petersdorf, R. G. (1983). An approach to infectious diseases. In R. G. Petersdorf, R. D. Adams, E. Braunwald, K. J. Isselbacher, J. B. Martin, & J. D. Wilson (Eds.), *Harrison's principle of internal medicine* (10th ed., pp. 831–843). New Delhi, India: McGraw Hill.

Pinkerton, H. (1971). Rickettsial, chlamydia and viral diseases. In W.A.D. Anderson (Ed.), *Pathology* (6th ed., Vol. 1, pp. 365–408). St. Louis, MO: C.V. Mosby Company.

Satoskar, R. S., & Bhandarkar, S. D. (1999). *Pharmacology and pharmacotherapeutics* (16th ed.). Bombay, India: Popular Prakashan.

chapter thirty

Tuberculosis

Basic concept of homeopathy – thirty

In tuberculosis, the killing of mycobacteria will kill the patient. If we could succeed today in putting a fluid into the economy that would destroy the bacteria that consumptive would soon die.

Argument

James Kent is another name, highly respected in the field of homeopathy. Lectures on homeopathic philosophy by James Kent are popular. Kent said in his lectures,

> Tubercles come first and the bacillus is secondary. It has never been found prior to the tubercle, but it follows that. Bacilli are not the cause of disease, they never come until after the disease … The bacteria theory would make it appear that the all wise Creator has sent these microorganisms to make man sick … Hahnemann did not adopt any such theory of bacteriology … If we could succeed today in putting a fluid into the economy that would destroy the bacteria that consumptive would soon die. (Kent, 1993, pp. 52–53)

Today we know with certainty that

> Tuberculosis is a specific infectious disease caused by a bacteria Mycobacterium tuberculosis. Tuberculosis chemotherapy has been one of the most significant advances during this century. With the evolution of controlled trials, the chemotherapy of tuberculosis is now more rationally based than in the treatment of other infectious diseases. The objective of chemotherapy treatment is cure, that is the elimination of both the fast and slowly multiplying bacilli from the patient's body. (Park, 1997, p. 265)

DOI: 10.1201/9781003228622-30

Kent says that the killing of *M. tuberculosis* will kill the patient. It means antibiotic or chemotherapeutic drugs, which kill the bacteria, will not cure the disease but will be responsible for death of patients. According to homeopathy, death will be increased by chemotherapeutic agents. Today we know that the above concept of Kent and Hahnemann is absolutely wrong.

Nowadays antituberculosis chemotherapy has reduced the mortality of tuberculosis patients. It is a major cause of death worldwide. If properly treated by drugs, it is curable in all cases, if drugs are not resistant. If untreated, the disease may be fatal within 5 years in 50–65% of cases. With the help of DOTS (case detection, short-course chemotherapy, monitoring), between 1995 and 2008, 36 million TB cases were cured and more than 6 million deaths were averted (Raviglione & Brien, 2012, p. 1340, 1358). Due to the use of antitubercular drugs, prognosis is excellent in primary pulmonary tuberculosis and its complications. Now fatal outcomes are extremely uncommon, even if the disease has reached an advanced stage.

Homeopathy rejects bacterial causes of disease but chemotherapeutic agents that kill bacteria are effective against diseases. Antibiotics are substances that kill microorganisms and "Approximately 30% of all hospitalized patients receive one or more courses of therapy with antibiotics and millions of potentially fatal infections have been cured" (Sande & Mandell, 1980, p. 1080).

Basics of homeopathy are wrong. Then derivations based on these basics will be definitely wrong. When we are sure that basic principles of homeopathy are wrong, then not a single disease can be cured by a homeopathic method of treatment. If some diseases are benefited by homeopathic drugs, then it is sure that there is either spontaneous recovery of the disease or placebo reaction.

Supporters of Ayurveda, homeopathy, and other nonscientific methods of treatment are actually responsible for many deaths of noneducated citizens specially villagers. Poor people and people from villages take Ayurveda and homeopathy and suffer a lot. Many people die or become disabled. Preventable diseases are spreading dangerously in India. I know many people who were taking Ayurvedic or homeopathic treatment for tuberculosis ultimately died. Many people first take medical treatment for one or two months, then start homeopathy or Ayurveda. Tuberculosis treatment should be taken 6–12 months continuously for complete treatment. Otherwise, the tuberculosis of these patients becomes resistant, and then it is not possible to treat them. Such foolishness is responsible for spreading many diseases like malaria and tuberculosis. "The emergence of drug resistant strains of microorganisms or parasites is promoted by treatments that do not result in cure" (Park, 1997, p. 265).

Chapter thirty: Tuberculosis 111

When MBBS doctors, who study pathology, diagnosis, and treatment of diseases, support Ayurveda and homeopathy, it proves that they do not know anything regarding medical science. In medical science, they read that microorganisms are responsible agents for many diseases but they support homeopathy that says microorganisms are never the cause of any disease. These experts also promote Ayurveda that has no pharmacokinetic and pharmacodynamic study, and which favors unwise etiology of diseases like dishonor of teacher is responsible for tuberculosis. These MBBS doctors create confusion in the society and they are mainly responsible for spreading preventable diseases and failure of WHO and Government Health Programme.

References

Kent, J. T. (1993). *Lectures on homeopathic philosophy*. Delhi, India: B. Jain Publishers.
Park, K. (1997). *Park's textbook of preventive and social medicine* (15th ed.). Jabalpur, India: Banarsidas Bhanot Publisher.
Raviglione, M. C., & Brien, R. J. O. (2012). Tuberculosis. In D. L. Long, D. L. Kasper, J. L. Jameson, A. S. Fauci, S. L. Hauser, & J. Loscalzo (Eds.), *Harrison's principles of internal medicine* (18th ed., Volume 1, pp. 1340–1359). New York, NY: McGraw Hill.
Sande, M. A., & Mandell, G. L. (1980). Antimicrobial agents: general consideration. In A. G. Gilman, L. Goodman, & A. Gilman (Eds.), *Goodman and Gilman's pharmacological basis of therapeutics* (6th ed., pp. 1080–1105). New York, NY: Macmillan.

chapter thirty one

One disease protects from another disease

Basic concept of homeopathy – thirty one

Kent said that persons suffering from diabetes, tuberculosis, and Bright's disease cannot suffer from other dissimilar mild infections like dysentery.

Argument

Kent has also said in his lectures,

> Dissimilar diseases can suspend another disease. He also said, if a person has some form of mild chronic disease, a severe attack of dysentery will cause that disease to disappear temporarily and the new disease will take hold and run its course and when it subsides the old symptoms will come back again. (Kent, 1993, p. 111)

According to his opinion, if the previous disease is strong, then subsequent disease, if dissimilar, cannot suppress the previous disease. Kent has mentioned some examples that were the basis of the above conclusions.

> A number of persons who are anything but strong are really invalids, one in consumption, another in the last stages of Bright's disease, another with diabetes. We call them all together and find that none of them have had dysentery or small pox or whatever disease was epidemic. (Kent, 1993, p. 11)

Kent said in his lectures that persons suffering from diabetes, tuberculosis, and Bright's disease cannot suffer from other dissimilar mild infections like dysentery and smallpox.

These observations are very important because homeopathy is based on these observations. If we can prove that these observations are wrong,

DOI: 10.1201/9781003228622-31

113

114   *Homeopathy*

then undoubtedly we can say that homeopathy is also wrong. Kent observed that patients with diabetes, tuberculosis, and Bright's disease cannot suffer from any other infection like dysentery or smallpox. But what are the facts? "Diabetic patients also suffer from diarrhoea" (Foster, 1983, p. 675). Other diseases having dissimilar symptomatology also exist with diabetes and it is against the rule of homeopathy that diseases of dissimilar symptomatology cannot exist together in a patient. Malignant external otitis and rhinocerebral mucormycosis, which are characterized by periorbital and perinasal swelling, pain, blood nasal discharge, and increased lacrimation, also exist with diabetes. Diabetes is characterized by thirst, polydipsia, polyuria, nocturia, tiredness, loss of weight, white marks on clothing, impotence, pruritus vulvae, and paresthesia or pain in limbs. Emphysematous cholecystitis is a variant of gallbladder disease that tends to affect diabetic men. Infestations of the skin with candida and dermatophytes are common and bacterial infections of a variety of types also occur (Foster, 1983, pp. 677–678).

Homeopathy says two similar diseases cannot exist in the body because one disease cures another disease of similar symptomatology. Homeopathy also says that two diseases of dissimilar symptomatology cannot exist together in the body because one disease will suspend another disease.

Tuberculosis and HIV have different symptomatology but both diseases may remain in a single patient together. What we observed, "Worldwide the number of people infected with both HIV and tuberculosis is rising. To make the global situation worse, tuberculosis has formed a lethal partnership with HIV" (Park, 1997, p. 150). This observation is against Kent's view that tuberculosis patients cannot suffer from other diseases.

HIV infection is associated with various diseases of similar and dissimilar symptomatology. Seventy percent of HIV-infected people experience fever, rash, and sore throat, a few weeks after the initial infection of HIV. Tuberculosis, Kaposi sarcoma, inflammation of retina in cytomegalovirus retinitis, dry, nonproductive cough, weight loss, fever in pneumocystis carinii pneumonia, mild hemiplegia and other neurological signs and symptoms in toxoplasma encephalitis, fever, headache, vomiting, neck stiffness in cryptococcal meningitis, pain and burning sensation, skin blisters in herpes zoster, and other skin infections are usually associated with HIV infection (Park, 1997, pp. 261–263).

What conclusion can be drawn by analyzing the above paragraph? Disease of similar and dissimilar symptomatology can exist together. If it is true, then the concept of homeopathy is wrong. Subclinical infections and latent infections confused Hahnemann and Kent. In subclinical cases,

> Disease agent may multiply in the host but does not manifest itself by signs and symptoms. Persons

Chapter thirty one: One disease protects from another disease 115

> who are thus sick are unknown to themselves and others ... barring a few e.g. measles, subclinical infection occurs in most infectious diseases. In some diseases e.g. rubella, mumps, polio, hepatitis A and B, Japanese encephalitis, influenza, diphtheria a great deal of subclinical infections occur frequently during a person's lifetime, they are responsible for the immunity. (Park, 1997, p. 84)

> In latent infection the host does not shed the infectious agent which lies dormant within the host without symptoms ... e.g. latent infection occurs in herpes simplex, Brill-Zinser disease, infections due to slow viruses, ancylostomiasis, etc. The role of latent infection in the perpetuation of certain infectious agents appears to be great. (Park, 1997, p. 84)

Hahnemann and Kent gave importance to symptoms only. They did not understand the presence of microbes inside the body. Whenever immunity weakens, subclinical infections manifest as signs and symptoms. If there are no symptoms, then they say that there is no disease. For example, viral infections produce interferon, an antiviral substance that also prevents further viral infection. If interferon is not in sufficient amounts, then there may be chances that a second subsequent infection may remain in subclinical form without producing signs and symptoms. Hahnemann may have observed in this case that the previous disease prevented the development of the second disease, but in fact second disease remained in subclinical form.

Hahnemann and Kent did not know about subclinical and latent infections that were also responsible for their wrong conclusions. Subclinical infections can be detected only by laboratory tests, e.g., antibody response, recovery of the organisms, skin sensitivity, and biochemical tests.

For analytical study, knowledge of subclinical infection and latent infection is important. Similarly, the concept of incubation period should be known to persons doing a study like Hahnemann. "An infection becomes apparent only after a certain incubation period which is defined as the time interval between invasion by an infectious agent and appearance of the first sign or symptoms of the disease" (Park, 1997, p. 88).

When the disease agent becomes in sufficient amounts, the disease becomes overt. Infective dose, portal of entry, and individual susceptibility determine incubation period. Incubation period varies for different infectious diseases and this also differs from one person to another. Incubation period is very short in cholera, bacillary dysentery, and influenza, e.g., – few hours to 2–3 days. In some diseases, it is 10 days to 3 weeks; examples are typhoid infection, chickenpox, measles, and mumps. There are also diseases that have weeks to months or years of incubation period. In these cases, accurate assessment of incubation period is very difficult. Cancer, heart disease, and mental illness also have incubation periods of months or years (Park, 1997, p. 88).

Now it should be clear in our mind that by only studying symptoms, it can never be possible to tell, "One disease cures another similar disease", which is the basic principle of homeopathy.

References

Foster, D. W. (1983). Diabetes mellitus. In R. G. Petersdorf, R. D. Adams, E. Braunwald, K. J. Isselbacher, J. B. Martin, & J. D. Wilson (Eds.), *Harrison's principle of internal medicine* (10th ed., pp. 661–679). New Delhi, India: McGraw Hill.

Kent, J. T. (1993). *Lectures on homeopathic philosophy.* Delhi, India: B. Jain Publishers.

Park, K. (1997). *Park's textbook of preventive and social medicine* (15th ed.). Jabalpur, India: Banarsidas Bhanot Publisher.

chapter thirty two

Therapeutic effectiveness

Basic concept of homeopathy – thirty two

In homeopathy, "To know the effectiveness of a drug, it should not be given to the patients", because in patients symptoms produced by drug and by disease will be mixed and then it will be difficult to separate. To know therapeutic effectiveness, drugs should be given to healthy persons. In severe acute and chronic diseases, which constitute by far the greater portion of all human ailments, crude nature is powerless, in these neither the vital force with its self-aiding faculty nor allopathy in imitation of it can affect a lysis.

Argument

Natural history of disease should be known for that person who discovers any new treatment. Without knowing the natural course, a claim of cure by a drug is useless. The study of the natural course of disease is not a part of any pathy. Normal observation of the natural course of a disease will remain the same irrespective of the type of pathy.

"As warts often disappear spontaneously, at any treatment which is in use that time will gain an undeserved reputation as a wart cure" (Rains & Ritchie, 1977, p. 101). "Proctitis is an inflammation of the rectal mucosa characterized by loss of blood in motions, often the complaint is one of diarrhoea, fortunately the condition is self limiting" (Rains & Ritchie, 1977, p. 1073). Most viral infections are self-limiting. Typhoid fever is also cured spontaneously when treatment is not given.

> The clinical manifestations and duration of illness vary markedly from one patient to another. Mild form of disease characterized primarily by fever may last only for a week or illness may be prolonged lasting 8 weeks or more if untreated. In a typical patient, not treated with antimicrobials, the illness lasts for about 4 weeks. (Guerrant & Hook, 1983, p. 959)

Almost all infectious diseases except few like rabies and HIV are spontaneously cured if sufficient immunity is in the body.

"In diabetic neuropathy, the most common picture is that of peripheral neuropathy, the symptoms include numbness, paresthesias,

DOI: 10.1201/9781003228622-32

118   *Homeopathy*

severe hyperesthesias and pain. The pain which may be deep seated and severe, is often worse at night. Fortunately extreme pain syndromes are usually self limited" (Foster, 1983, p. 675). Low-back pain usually recovers spontaneously. Although its causes are poorly understood, it is improved with the body's own healing power. Most patients with back pain will usually and rapidly recover even when their pain is severe. This prognosis is true regardless of treatment method or even without treatment (Deyo, 1998, pp. 49–50).

Alternative systems are widely used in cervical and back pain. In acute low back pain without radiculopathy (injury to nerve), full recovery can be expected in patients without leg pain. The prognosis is excellent. Spontaneous improvement can mislead clinicians about the efficacy of treatment interventions. Perhaps as a result, many ineffective treatments have become popular in the past. Back pain is the most common reason for seeking complementary and alternative treatments. A common cause of back pain is a herniated disk with nerve root impingement resulting in back pain with radiation down the leg. The prognosis of this condition is generally favorable. As with low back pain, spontaneous improvement is the norm for acute neck pain and the symptomatic relief while natural healing processes proceed (Engstrom & Deyo, 2012).

"Most fevers are associated with self-limited infections, such as common viral diseases" (Dinarello & Porat, 2008, p. 120). In lobar pneumonia patients, without treatment, resolution occurs on the eight day. Complete resolution and regeneration take from one to three weeks. Since there is no tissue destruction in lobar pneumonia, the lung parenchyma returns to normal (Heath & Kay, 1976, p. 414).

A study of skin diseases plays a very important role in the analysis of principles of homeopathy. According to homeopathy, suppression of skin diseases by external applications of drugs redirects the diseases internally and creates internal diseases. But in fact the cure of skin diseases has no relation with the development of internal disease. Many skin diseases are resolved spontaneously which confuse Hahnemann who wrongly thought that treatment of skin diseases by external means creates internal pathology. "Alopecia areata is a common condition characterised by a patchy loss of hair without atrophy … It may affect any hairy area of the body and is usually reversible" (Wadhwa et al., 2008, p. 900). Staphylococcal scalded skin syndrome (SSSS) occurs mainly in infants and children under the age of five years. The most common cause of SSSS is *Staphylococcus aureus*. In this disease, rapid recovery is the rule. Healing takes place in one to two weeks even in the absence of treatment. But in untreated cases, a mortality of 2–3% is present (Singh et al., 2008, pp. 233–234).

Dermatophytosis is a superficial fungal infection of keratinized tissue. The infection is commonly known as tinea. The fungal growth rate

Chapter thirty two: Therapeutic effectiveness 119

must either equal or exceed the epidermal turnover rate, as otherwise the organism will be shade quickly. The infection spontaneously resolves. If a second infection by the same organism is produced, the site becomes inflamed very early and resolves relatively quickly (Kanwar & De, 2008, pp. 252–254). Warts are benign proliferation of the skin resulting from infection with human papillomavirus. Warts occur at any age. Most cutaneous warts are self-limiting and spontaneously regress within two years of onset. About 65% of common warts disappear spontaneously within two years. The regression is earlier in male children. Regression of common warts is asymptomatic and occurs gradually over several weeks usually without any sequelae (Criton, 2008, pp. 366–370).

Molluscum contagiosum is a viral infection of skin caused by poxvirus, a virus, affecting children and sexually active adults. It is not always necessary to treat all cases since it resolves spontaneously (Criton, 2008, pp. 333–334). Herpes simplex is a virus infection distributed worldwide. It involves mainly the orofacial and genital site. Antiviral treatment is not necessary for mild uncomplicated herpes simplex infection (Criton, 2008, pp. 337–343). Acute varicella (chickenpox) is a self-limited disease characterized by fever, malaise, and a generalized pruritic rash. Varicella is typically a benign self-limiting infection in healthy children (Criton, 2008, pp. 344–346). Most patients recover from herpes zoster without any complications (Criton, 2008, p. 349).

Pityriasis rosea is an acute self-limiting disorder with a very characteristic skin rash mainly involving children and young adults. The treatment is essentially symptomatic. Most importantly, a patient should be reassured regarding the self-limiting nature of the rash (Criton, 2008, pp. 375–377).

Now it can be said that various skin diseases tend to recover spontaneously which confuses Hahnemann. Herpes zoster spontaneously resolves in three to four weeks, chickenpox in three to four weeks; pityriasis rosea, a papulosquamous disease which recovers in six to seven weeks; pityriasis alba – a kind of eczematous disorder in which children get hypopigmented spots usually disappears after puberty. Acne vulgaris usually disappears after the age of 25 years. Alopecia areata is the commonest cause of patchy hair loss. It is a self-limiting disease. It usually recovers in four to six months. Majority of the cases having infective dermatosis also tend to recover even if no treatment is given. Patients having pyoderma, dermatophyte infection, and candidiasis tend to improve with the onset of winter without any treatment. Herpes simplex usually disappears in one to two weeks but the virus may reactivate again in a few patients. Facial warts may disappear in most of cases without any treatment in three to six months. Molluscum contagiosum can disappear in more than 50% cases without treatment in three to six months.

"Erysipelas, a specific form of cellulitis caused by beta hemolytic streptococci ... Usually within a week or ten days there is spontaneous remission, and shortly thereafter complete healing occurs" (Hoppes, 1971, p. 286).

Carcinomas are malignant tumors and obviously are of clinical importance because of the extensive mortality and morbidity they produce. Most cancers are treated by surgery. Radiotherapy and drug therapy are also part of cancer therapy. It is the general concept of the public that if a person is suffering from cancer, he will die or require extensive surgical or nonsurgical treatment. Nobody thinks that cancer may resolve spontaneously but medical reports say that cancer may resolve spontaneously.

> Certainly there is an interplay of tumor-host relationship so that all factors combine to determine the ultimate biological behaviour of the neoplasm. Benign tumors not only grow slowly but also at times reach a point where they seem to become dormant or even to regress. This is true e.g. with leiomyomas of the uterus, which often cease growing after the menopause occasionally even malignant tumors enter a stage of dormancy and in rare but well documented instances, they may regress spontaneously. (Meissner & Warren, 1971, p. 551)

"In malignant melanoma clinically spontaneous regression often heralded by sudden onset of irregular halo around tumour" (Rossi, 1996, p. 259). Tumors are divided into two groups, one is relatively innocuous tumors designated as benign and the other more rapidly growing, dangerous and destructive tumors known as malignant. The synonym of malignant tumor is cancer. Benign tumors have no metastases and very little tissue destruction while cancer has widespread metastases and much tissue destruction. "Ganglioneuroma is a benign tumor of neurological tissue while neuroblastoma is a malignant tumor. As a rare but remarkable event, neuroblastoma may undergo a form of self cure by maturing into a ganglioneuroma" (Lennox, 1976, p. 302) or "may regress spontaneously" (Blossom et al., 1997, p. 966). "Choriocarcinoma is a highly malignant tumour. In some instances removal of primary tumour has been followed by apparently spontaneous disappearance of metastasis" (Lennox, 1976, p. 307).

It is also known to medical science that diseases have variable natural history.

> Most diseases tend to wax and wane in severity, some disappear spontaneously with time, even malignant

Chapter thirty two: Therapeutic effectiveness 121

> neoplasm may undergo spontaneous remissions.
> A good experimental design must take into account
> the natural history of the disease under study by
> evaluating a large enough population of subjects
> over a sufficiently long period of time. (Berkowitz,
> 2004, p. 68)

We also know by normal observations that diseases have normal fluctuations. These normal fluctuations and presence of other diseases may influence the result of clinical study. To obtain accurate results,

> a cross over design which consists of alternating
> periods of administration of test drug, placebo
> preparation and standard drug control in each sub-
> ject. These sequences are systematically varied so
> that different subsets of patients receive each of the
> possible sequences of treatment. (Berkowitz, 2004,
> pp. 68–69)

There is also a psychological effect on patients. Even if an inert mate-rial is given to patients, most patients tend to respond in a positive way. It is known as placebo response and this may also involve objective bio-chemical, pathological change, and also a change in complaint of patients associated with disease.

> The magnitude of the response varies considerably
> from patient to patient. However the incidence of the
> placebo response is fairly constant being observed
> in 20 to 40% of patients in almost all studies. Placebo
> toxicity also occurs but usually involves subjec-
> tive effects of stomach upset, insomnia, sedation.
> (Berkowitz, 2004, p. 69)

This full method of studying drug clinically is known as double blind placebo controlled cross over design.

> Enormous costs from $100/- million to over
> $500 million (dollar) are involved in the develop-
> ment of a single successful new drug. These costs
> include the labour invested in searching for useful
> new molecules. 5000–10000 may be synthesized for
> each successful new drug introduced and the costs

of detailed basic and clinical studies and promotion of the ultimate candidate molecule. (Berkowitz, 2001, p. 64)

Now we should know how much time will be taken by a drug for its development? And what types of studies are required before successful development of a drug or treatment? Initial safety, biological effects, receptor study, enzyme inhibition and selectivity, drug absorption, metabolism, excretion, therapeutic efficacy, dose range, kinetics and adverse reaction, acute, subacute, chronic studies, effect on reproductive behavior, carcinogenic potential, mutagenic potential are studied and analyzed by clinical pharmacologist and physicians. Most new drug candidates are identified through chemical modification of known molecules, screening of natural products or previously discovered chemical entities for biological activity or rational drug design based on an understanding of biological mechanisms. Average ten years are taken by a drug before marketing and even after marketing surveillance is continued. If new toxicity appears after marketing, the drug is withdrawn from the market and the whole exercise of drug development becomes useless.

Conclusively it can be said. "Doctors who think they can assess the value of a treatment by using it on patients in an uncontrolled fashion have the whole history of therapeutics against them" (Laurence & Bennett, 1987, p. 49). To know the therapeutic efficacy of a drug, it should be given to patients and after controlled trials and statistical analysis, we can say about the effectiveness of a drug or treatment. Drug is given to healthy volunteers to know pharmacokinetic character and adverse effects of a drug. But in homeopathy to know the effectiveness of a drug, it should not be given to patients because in patients symptoms produced by drug and by disease will be mixed and then it will be difficult to separate them (Hahnemann, 1921/1996, p. 120). In homeopathy, drugs are never studied in patients. Drugs are given to healthy persons and symptoms produced by drugs are recorded. If the drug produces the same symptoms in healthy persons as the disease itself, then that drug is considered to be the best treatment for that disease.

Hahnemann was a highly intelligent person but he suffered from lack of accurate information. The capacity of analyzing, capacity of invention, creation, and research ability indicate intelligence. Knowledge is a collection of information. A highly intelligent person cannot tell the truth if he has wrong information. A highly advanced computer will give wrong conclusions if we feed wrong or incomplete information. Hahnemann worked from 1810 to 1842. At that time, sufficient information regarding health and disease was not available. This is the cause why Hahnemann made the wrong conclusion.

Chapter thirty two: Therapeutic effectiveness 123

Hahnemann said two things very accurately. He should be appreciated for this. First he said that old allopathy is dangerous and detrimental to the human body. Hahnemann writes accurately.

> Although there previously never was a drop of blood too much in the living human body yet the old school practitioners consider an imaginary excess of blood as the main material cause of all haemorrhage and inflammations which they must remove and drain off by venesections, cupping and leeches. In general inflammatory fevers, in acute pleurisy they even regard the coagulable lymph in the blood ... which they endeavor to get rid of if possible by repeated venesections. (Hahnemann, 1921/1993, pp. 39–40)

"They thus often bleed the patient nearly to death" (Hahnemann, 1921/1993, p. 39–40). Second statement is correctly said by Hahnemann regarding natural recovery of some diseases. Hahnemann said, "It is only the slighter and acute diseases that tend when the natural period of their course has expired to terminate quietly in resolution, as it is called with or without the employment of not very aggressive allopathic remedies" (Hahnemann, 1921/1993, p. 52).

Hahnemann agreed that some diseases resolved spontaneously. But Hahnemann made the mistake by presuming that severe acute and chronic diseases cannot resolve automatically. As Hahnemann said,

> In severe acute and chronic diseases which constitute by far the greater portion of all human ailments, crude nature and the old school are equally powerless, in these neither the vital force with its self aiding faculty nor allopathy in imitation if it, can affect a lyses, but at the most a mere temporary truce during which the enemy fortifies himself, in order sooner or later to recommence the attack with still greater violence. (Hahnemann, 1921/1993, p. 52)

It was a great mistake by Hahnemann. Many severe acute and chronic diseases also resolve automatically. This fact was not known to Hahnemann and this is mainly responsible for development of an inaccurate system of treatment that is homeopathy.

References

Berkowitz, B. A. (2001). Basic and clinical evaluation of new drugs. In B. G. Katzung (Ed.), *Basic and clinical pharmacology* (8th ed., pp. 64–74). New York, NY: McGraw Hill (A Lange Medical Book).

Berkowitz, B. A. (2004). Basic and clinical evaluation of new drugs. In B. G. Katzung (Ed.), *Basic and clinical pharmacology* (9th ed., pp. 64–74). Boston, MA: McGraw Hill (A Lange Medical Book).

Blossom, G. B., Stronger, Z., & Stephenson, L. W. (1997). Neoplasm of the mediastinum. In V. Devita Jr, S. Hellman, & S. A. Rosenberg (Eds.), *Cancer: Principles and practice of oncology* (5th ed., pp. 951–970). Philadelphia, PA: Lippincott-Raven.

Criton, S. (2008). Viral infection. In R. G. Valia, & Ameet, R. Valia (Eds.), *IADVL textbook of dermatology* (3rd ed., Vol. 1, pp. 331–396). Mumbai, India: Bhalani Publishing House.

Deyo, R. A. (1998). Low-back pain. *Scientific American, 279*(2), 48–53.

Dinarello, C. A., & Porat, R. (2008). Fever and hyperthermia. In A. S. Fauci, D. L. Kasper, D. L. Longo, E. Braunwald, S. L. Hauser, & J. L. Jameson (Eds.), *Harrison's principle of internal medicine* (17th ed., pp. 117–121). New York, NY: McGraw Hill.

Engstrom, J. W., & Deyo, R. A. (2012). Back and neck pain. In D. L. Longo, D. L. Kasper, J. L. Jameson, A. S. Fauci, S. L. Hauser, & J. Loscalzo (Eds), *Harrison's principles of internal medicine* (18th ed., Vol. 1, pp. 129–142). New York, NY: McGraw Hill.

Foster, D. W. (1983). Diabetes mellitus. In R. G. Petersdorf, R. D. Adams, E. Braunwald, K. J. Isselbacher, J. B. Martin, & J. D. Wilson (Eds.), *Harrison's principle of internal medicine* (10th ed., pp. 661–679). New York, NY: McGraw Hill.

Guerrant, R. L., & Hook, E. (1983). Salmonella infection. In R. G. Petersdorf, R. D. Adams, E. Braunwald, K. J. Isselbacher, J. B. Martin, & J. D. Wilson (Eds.), *Harrison's principle of internal medicine* (10th ed., pp. 957–965). New York, NY: McGraw Hill.

Hahnemann, S. (1993). *Organon of medicine* (6th ed.) (W. Boericke, Trans.). New Delhi, India: B. Jain Publishers. (Original work published in 1921).

Hahnemann, S. (1996). *Organon of medicine* (6th ed.) (P. Devi, Trans). New Delhi, India: B. Jain Publishers. (Original book published in 1921).

Heath, D., & Kay, J. M. (1976). Respiratory system. In J. R. Anderson (Ed.), *Muir's textbook of pathology* (10th ed., pp. 378–449). London, United Kingdom: ELBS & Edward Arnold.

Hoppes, H., C. (1971). Bacterial diseases. In W. A. D. Anderson (Ed.), *Pathology* (6th ed., Vol. 1, pp. 270–372.).St. Louis, MO: C.V. Mosby Company.

Kanwar, A. J., & De, D. (2008). Superficial fungal infections. In R. G. Valia, & Ameet R Valia (Eds.), *IADVL textbook of dermatology* (3rd ed., Vol. 1, pp. 252–297). Mumbai, India: Bhalani Publishing House.

Laurence, D. R., & Bennett, P. N. (1987). *Clinical pharmacology* (6th ed.). Harlow, United Kingdom: ELBS and Churchill Livingstone.

Lennox, B. (1976). Tumours three, other varieties. In J. R. Anderson (Ed.), *Muir's textbook of pathology* (10th ed., pp. 289–309). London, United Kingdom: ELBS and Edward Arnold.

Chapter thirty two: Therapeutic effectiveness 125

Meissner, W. A., & Warren, S. (1971). Neoplasms. In W.A.D. Anderson (Ed.), *Pathology* (6th ed., Vol. 1, pp. 529–561). St. Louis, MO: C.V. Mosby Company.

Rains, A. J. H., & Ritchie, H. D. (1977). *Bailey and Love's short practice of surgery* (17th ed.). London, United Kingdom: H. K. Levi's and Co Ltd.

Rossi, J. (1996). *Ackerman's surgical pathology* (8th ed., Vol. 1). Singapore: Harcourt Brace and Company.

Singh, G., Kaur, V., & Singh, S. (2008). Bacterial infections. In R. G. Valia, & Ameet R Valia (Eds.). *IADVL textbook of dermatology* (3rd ed., Vol. 1, pp. 223–251). Mumbai, India: Bhalani Publishing House.

Wadhwa, S. L., Khopkar, U., & Nischal, K. C. (2008). Hair and scalp disorders. In R. G. Valia & Ameet R Valia (Eds.), *IADVL textbook of dermatology* (3rd ed., Vol. 1, pp. 864–948). Mumbai, India: Bhalani Publishing House.

chapter thirty three

Bright's disease and syphilis

Basic concept of homeopathy – thirty three

Kent concluded that one chronic disease (syphilis) suppressed another chronic disease (Bright's disease) and when syphilis was cured, Bright's disease again appeared. Then Kent said, "Dissimilars are unable to cure, they can only suppress".

Argument

Kent's lectures on homeopathic philosophy have been accepted as authorized documents. Kent said in his lecture,

> A patient is in the earlier stage of Bright's disease and the symptoms are clear enough to make a diagnosis. He takes syphilis and at once the kidney disease is held in abeyance, the albumin disappears from the urine and his waxiness is lost. But after a year's careful prescribing, the syphilitic state disappears and very soon the albumin appears again in the urine, the dropsy returns and he dies of an ordinary attack of Bright's disease. (Kent, 1993, p. 111)

This patient had three stages: (a) Patient suffered from edema and albuminuria in the first stage, which was said to be Bright's disease. (b) At the next stage, when syphilis appeared, Bright's disease was cured. (c) In the last stage, after one year, when syphilis was resolved, Bright's disease again reappeared and the patient died. Then Kent said, "Dissimilar are unable to cure, they can only suppress" (Kent, 1993, p. 111).

The conclusion that one disease suppresses another dissimilar chronic disease on the basis of above observation was wrong. What is Bright's disease, "Any one of a group of kidney disease attending with albuminuria and oedema known as Bright's disease" (Dorland, 1965). And what are the symptoms of nephritic syndrome? Acute nephritic syndrome consists of the abrupt onset of hematuria, proteinuria, azotemia, reduced GFR, hypertension, and edema. Nephritic syndrome is also included in Bright's disease. Within a week or so of onset, most patients

DOI: 10.1201/9781003228622-33

127

with postinfectious acute glomerulonephritis will begin to experience spontaneous resolution of hypertension and fluid retention (Brenner, 1983, p. 1632). "In cases of acute post-streptococcal glomerulonephritis, all experience a spontaneous resolution of abnormal clinical signs within a week after the onset of illness. Abnormalities in the urinary sediment and protein excretion subside slowly in the ensuing months. In a few cases several years elapse before the urinary sediment becomes consistently normal" (Brenner, 1983, p. 1633). "In many instances nephritic syndrome will abate following cure of the infection or withdrawal of the offending medication" (Brenner, 1983, p. 1640) and we know that various infections are self-limiting due to body immunity.

Today we also know, "Syphilis itself causes nephritic syndrome which is also characterized by albuminuria, hypoalbuminemia and edema" (Brenner, 1983, p. 1635). "In secondary syphilis renal involvement is associated with proteinuria" (Holmes, 1983, p. 1038).

"A few patients with syphilis develop the nephritic syndrome" (Anderson, 1976, p. 807).

Now we coordinate all the above statements. Kent said that the development of syphilis suppresses Bright's disease and later on after the treatment of syphilis, Bright's disease reappears and patients die. But what was the fact? The fact can be explained. Bright's disease of this patient must have been a part of secondary syphilis. First, there was an appearance of Bright's disease followed by other manifestations of syphilis. Some manifestations may dominate in one person, while other manifestations may dominate in another person. "The secondary lesions of syphilis subside within 2 to 6 weeks and the patient enters the latent stage" (Holmes, 1983, p. 1036). After a gap of one year, there was again the appearance of a late benign stage of syphilis. In this stage, gumma is produced, which may be multiple or diffuse. By gumma "any organ may be involved and about one fourth die as a result of tertiary syphilis" (Holmes, 1983, p 1039). The earlier part of disease must have been a type of Bright's disease, which was cured spontaneously. And the second and third parts of disease were definitely the secondary and tertiary stages of syphilis. Patient died due to kidney lesions of tertiary syphilis. Syphilis also causes renal involvement and further causes proteinuria and hematuria. Hahnemann wrongly understood two different diseases: syphilis and Bright's disease. Therefore, he made a mistake and formulated the wrong concept. Now we can say that by only studying symptoms without studying other aspects of disease and and proper diagnosis and evaluation, nothing can be said. If somebody says empirically, then it will definitely not be correct as Kent and Hahnemann said.

Chapter thirty three: Bright's disease and syphilis   129

References

Anderson, J. R. (1976). Urinary system. In J. R. Anderson (Ed.), *Muir's textbook of pathology* (10th ed., pp. 745–809). London, United Kingdom: ELBS and Edward Arnold.

Brenner, B. M. (1983). Major glomerulopathies. In R. G. Petersdorf, R. D. Adams, E. Braunwald, K. J. Isselbacher, J. B. Martin, & J. D. Wilson (Eds.), *Harrison's principle of internal medicine* (10th ed., pp. 1632–1642). New Delhi, India: McGraw Hill.

Dorland, W. A. N. (1965). *Dorland's medical dictionary.* London, United Kingdom: W.B. Saunders Company.

Holmes, K. K. (1983). Syphilis. In R. G. Petersdorf, R. D. Adams, E. Braunwald, K. J. Isselbacher, J. B. Martin, & J. D. Wilson (Eds.), *Harrison's principle of internal medicine* (10th ed., pp. 1034–1045). New Delhi, India: McGraw Hill.

Kent, J. T. (1993). *Lectures on homeopathic philosophy.* Delhi, India: B. Jain Publishers.

chapter thirty four

Fistula in ano

Basic concept of homeopathy – thirty four

Homeopathy condemns in principle the removal of external manifestations of disease by an external means.

Argument

"The Organon condemns in principle the removal of external manifestations of disease by an external means whatever" (Kent, 1993, p. 63). For the support of this statement, Kent gives the example of fistula in ano. Kent writes,

> The closure of that fistulous opening but If a patient is threatened with phthisis or is a weak patient, the closure of that fistulous opening of anus will throw him into a flame of excitement and will cause his death in a year or two ... The fistulous opening came there because it was of use ... When the patient is cured the fistulous opening ceases to be of use, the necessity for it to remain open has ceased and it heals up by itself. (Kent, 1993, p. 63)

Generalization should not have been made by Kent and Hahnemann from a single or a few observations. External outlets are must where pus is collected. Pus should be removed. If pus is not removed, then it is very difficult to get cured. In fistula in ano, "The fistula continues to discharge and because of constant reinfection from the anal canal or rectum, seldom if ever close permanently without surgical aid" (Rains & Ritchie, 1977, p. 1078). Fistula in ano has varied etiology like tuberculosis, ulcerative proctocolitis, Crohn's disease, bilharziasis, and lymphogranuloma inguinale. This varied etiology and continuous contamination and accumulation of pus require the evacuation of pus and treatment of a specific cause. Today we know, "About 2-3% of fistula in patients are tuberculous. The fistula will usually respond to antitubercular drugs" (Rains & Ritchie, 1977, p. 1080).

DOI: 10.1201/9781003228622-34

But generalization should not be made that external symptoms should not be managed. Homeopathy does not accept the concept of externally localized independent disease. According to this pathy, all localized external lesions are actually parts of internal disease. This pathy also opposes the treatment of external lesions by external means. When a localized lesion is a part of generalized internal disease, then in such cases, external localized treatment may not be effective, then internal disease has to be treated, e.g., syphilis and gonorrhea. But when external lesions are not parts of generalized disease, then external management has to be used. Today we know that various diseases are externally localized lesions, and these are not parts of internal generalized diseases; these are treated effectively by external means. Cyst, sinuses, sebaceous cyst, papilloma of skin, molluscum fibrosum, molluscum sebaceum, basal cell carcinoma of the skin, squamous cell carcinoma of skin, chalazion, cataract, conjunctivitis, cleft lip, cleft palate, neoplasms of the lip, boils, carbuncle, hyperplastic gingivitis, neoplasms of the breast, etc. are the localized external pathological lesions that can be managed only by external localized means. These lesions are independent and localized.

In the above examples, external manifestations are removed by external therapeutic methods, which indicate the homeopathic concept of opposition to external treatment is wrong.

References

Kent, J. T. (1993). *Lectures on homeopathic philosophy*. Delhi, India: B. Jain Publishers.
Rains, A. J. H., & Ritchie, H. D. (1977). *Bailey and Love's short practice of surgery* (17th ed.). London, United Kingdom: H. K. Levis and Co Ltd.

chapter thirty five

No organ can make the body sick

Basic concept of homeopathy – thirty five

No organ can make the body sick. Man is prior to his organs. Parts of the body can be removed and yet man will exist.

Argument

Kent writes, "It is great folly for a man to look into the organs themselves for the purpose of establishing a theory to find out whether the stomach makes the man sick or whether the stomach makes the liver sick and such like" (Kent, 1993, p. 54). Kent also writes, "No organ can make the body sick, man is prior to his organs, parts of the body can be removed and yet man will exist. There is no such thing as one organ making another sick" (Kent, 1993, p. 55).

Kent says that no organ can make the body sick, but what is reality? Delirium is characterized by clouding of consciousness, perceptual disturbances, incoherent speech, altered psychomotor activity, disorientation, memory impairment, and variability of clinical pictures from time to time. And delirium is produced by the pathology of specific organs. Pathology in the brain, pituitary, pancreas, adrenal, parathyroid, thyroid, liver, kidney, lung, and heart can produce delirium. Any one of the above organs can develop delirium if pathology occurs (Wells, 1985, pp. 842–844). This means, a person suffering from delirium indicates sickness.

Body can become sick when the lung, liver, heart, kidney, or any other organ of the body is damaged. Liver disorder creates hepatic coma. Kidney failure is responsible for death. Heart failure also damages the whole body. Heart attack is the main cause of death. When pathology or disease in one organ can cause death, then how Kent can say that damage or disease of one organ cannot make the body sick. Now we can say this statement of Kent is also wrong.

Kent further says, parts of the body can be removed and yet man will exist. How a man can survive when his liver, heart, both lungs, both kidneys, or brain are removed. A man can never survive when his vital organs are removed. Only a brainless person can say that a man can survive without a brain.

DOI: 10.1201/9781003228622-35

134 Homeopathy

Kent also said, "One organ cannot make another organ sick". But the whole medical knowledge says that one damaged organ always damages the other organ. I am giving a few examples. Chronic obstructive lung disease is a disease of the lung. After sometime, this disease damages the heart, which is labeled as cor pulmonale. Cancer of one organ affects various organs of the body by metastasis. "Carcinoma in the kidney affects adrenal gland, bone, brain, heart, lung, liver, lymph node, ovary, pancreas, skin, spleen, thyroid gland and muscles" (Lee, 1976, p. 538). Similarly, cancer of many organs can affect other organs of the body. Disease of the pancreas gives rise to diabetes mellitus. Diabetes of prolonged duration damages the kidney, eye, and nervous system. Damage in the brain also causes damage to other organs of the body. Brain controls all functions of the body. Damage in the brain leads to hemiplegia, paraplegia, vision loss, speech loss, etc. Hemiplegia means paralysis of half of the body, and paraplegia means paralysis of both the lower limbs. Conclusively, Kent was again wrong in his observations.

References

Kent, J. T. (1993). *Lectures on homeopathic philosophy.* Delhi, India: B. Jain Publishers.

Lee, F. D. (1976). Alimentary tract. In J. R. Anderson (Ed.), *Muir's textbook of pathology* (10th ed., pp. 530–600). London, United Kingdom: ELBS and Edward Arnold.

Wells, C. E. (1985). Organic syndromes: Delirium. In H. I. Kaplan, & B. J. Sadock (Eds.), *Comprehensive textbook of psychiatry* (4th ed., pp. 838–851). Baltimore, MD: Williams and Wilkins.

chapter thirty six

Bacteria are harmless

Basic concept of homeopathy – thirty six

Hahnemann reached the conclusion that it is not from external things that man becomes sick, not from bacteria, nor environment but from causes in himself. He said that intravenous administration of fluid is dangerous to the body, and bacteria have not been sent on earth to destroy man. Bacteria are perfectly harmless in every respect.

Argument

Kent and Hahnemann say again and again, "It is not from external things that man becomes sick, not from bacteria nor environment but from causes in himself" (Kent, 1993, p. 34). Hahnemann derived this conclusion on the basis of some results mentioned by some contemporary experts. (a) A girl in Glasgow, eight years of age, having been bit by a mad dog, the surgeon immediately cut that part and cleaned out, and yet 36 days afterward, she was seized with hydrophobia that killed her in 2 days. (b) Life was endangered by injecting a little pure water into a vein. (c) Even the mildest fluids introduced into the vein endangered life (Hahnemann, 1921/2017, pp. 13–15).

In example one, Hahnemann observed that after a dog bite, part was cleaned and removed from the body still the patient suffered from hydrophobia and died. That's why he concluded that external microorganisms were not responsible for hydrophobia and death. Then he presumed that the cause of hydrophobia was within the person and not related to dog bite. Truth was missed by Hahnemann. But it was the reality. Rabies, also known as hydrophobia, is an acute highly fatal viral disease of the central nervous system. It is transmitted to man by bites or licks of rabid animals. Rabies virus spreads from the site of infection via the peripheral nerves toward the central nervous system. Bite wounds should not be immediately sutured to prevent extra trauma, which may help spread the virus into the deeper tissues (Park, 1997, pp. 207–210). In this example, dissection at the site of dog bite exposed nerve endings that facilitated virus transmission to the central nervous system. "Once the virus reaches the central nervous system, it replicates almost exclusively within the gray matter and then passes centrifugally

DOI: 10.1201/9781003228622-36

135

along autonomic nerves to reach other tissue" (Corey, 1983, p. 1136), causing death.

In example two, Hahnemann studied observations of other physicians and found that intravenous administration of fluid is dangerous to the body. But this observation was absolutely wrong. Today drugs and fluids are routinely administered intravenously and the lives of crores of patients are being saved. Cefotaxime, ampicillin, gentamicin, ciprofloxacin, metronidazole, aminophylline, corticosteroids, morphine derivatives, electrolytes, water, and saline are also administered intravenously, and patients get benefit. Intravenous administration of a substance is not dangerous to life.

Regarding air administration, Hahnemann's opinion was correct. Air administration in circulation is dangerous to life and may cause death. All substances cannot be administered intravenously, it is correct. Intravenous route increased risk of adverse effects. It is not suitable for oily solutions. Drugs should be in aqueous solution to administer by intravenous route. Insoluble substances, if administered by intravenous route, damage the body and may cause death.

In the above examples, Hahnemann wanted to say, "The causes of our maladies cannot be material since the least foreign material substance, however mild it may appear to us, if introduced into our blood vessels is promptly ejected by vital force, as though it were a poison or when this does not happen death ensues" (Hahnemann, 1921/1993, p. 44). But Hahnemann's conclusion was wrong and observations of respective physicians, who said intravenous fluid administration causes death, were also wrong.

Kent also writes,

> The bacteria are results of disease. Microscopical little fellows are not the disease cause but that they come after that. They are scavengers accompanying the disease and that they are perfectly harmless in every respect. They are the outcome of the disease, are present wherever the disease is and by the microscope it has been discovered that every pathological result has its corresponding bacteria. (Kent,1993, p. 22)

Kent also said,

> Bacteria have a use for there is nothing in the whole world that does not have a use and there is nothing sent on earth to destroy man. The bacteria theory

Chapter thirty six: Bacteria are harmless   *137*

would make it appear that the all wise creator has
sent these microorganisms here to make man sick.
Hahnemann did not adopt any such theory as
bacteriology. (Kent, 1993, p. 52)

Kent also writes, "Cause of phthisis is not in the bacteria but in the
virus which the bacteria are sent to destroy. Man lives longer with the
bacteria than he would without them" (Kent, 1993, p. 53).

Today it has been proved that bacteria are the cause of many diseases
like tuberculosis, leprosy, typhoid, dysentery, meningitis, gonorrhea, and
respiratory tract infection. If somebody still accepts the view that bacteria
are not responsible for any disease, then we can say that he does not know
anything regarding medical science. The same statement is true for those
who believe in homeopathy.

In support of the view that bacteria are not responsible for any disease, Kent writes,

A dissecting wound is very serious, if the body dis-
sected is recently dead and this we would suppose to
be due to some bacteria of wonderful power capable
of establishing such dreadful erysipelatous poisoning that would go into man's blood and strike him
down with a sort of septicaemia. In truth, soon after
death we have a ptomaine poison, the dead body poison, which is alkaloid in character but we have not
yet discovered the presence of bacteria. The poison
is there and if a man pricks himself while dissecting that body and does not take care of the wound
he may have a serious illness and die. But if after
the cadaver has remained sometime and become
infected with bacteria, the dissector pricks himself
the wound is not dangerous. (Kent, 1993, p. 52)

Kent did not agree that erysipelas infection was due to bacteria. Kent
was of the opinion that after death, there is production of ptomaine poison in the dead body, which is fatal to living beings, and bacteria are not
related to the production of this ptomaine poison. Kent also said that after
death, the body was infected with bacteria but these bacteria were not
harmful to the body because bacteria from cadaver did not make wounds
dangerous. All these conclusions of Kent were wrong. It has been proved
that "Erysipelas is an acute infection of the skin and subcutaneous tissue
caused by group A streptococci, other streptococci and even staphylococci
and pneumococci" (Bison, 1983, p. 932). These all organisms are bacteria

138   *Homeopathy*

and responsible for erysipelas diseases. Kent did not know regarding ptomaine poison, how it is produced, and in what amount it is dangerous. Today we know,

> Ptomaines are alkaloidal bodies produced by the action of saprophytic microorganisms upon nitrogenous materials, probably during the process of decomposition. They are called cadaveric alkaloids as they are generated in the dead tissue while alkaloids secreted by the living cells during the metabolic processes are called leucomaines. Most of the ptomaines that have been discovered are non-poisonous except neurine and mydaleine which are actively poisonous and produce symptoms resembling those produced by atropine, muscarine, aconite. It is said that neurine is not generated till the fifth or sixth day has elapsed since death and mydaleine not until the seventh day and that too in traces only. (Modi, 1975, p. 631)

Usually ptomaines are nonpoisonous and poisonous ptomaine are only two in number. These poisonous ptomaines are produced in very small amounts, and by dissecting instruments, the amount that is transferred from dead body to living tissue is very less likely to produce toxic symptomatology in healthy persons. Ptomaines are produced by bacteria. Again, Kent was wrong about the statement that he gave for ptomaines.

Kent also writes, bacteria present in cadaver are not harmful because they do not make wounds dangerous, that's why Kent makes the conclusion that bacteria cannot produce any disease or any harm to human beings. But Kent was always wrong. He could not understand facts due to a lack of available knowledge. Why bacteria from cadaver cannot produce disease in healthy human beings? Here is the explanation.

> Clostridium welchii, Clostridium oedematiens and Clostridium septicum are three most important anaerobic sporulating bacteria. Being anaerobic and saprophytic, they cannot multiply in living oxygenated tissue but they flourish in dead tissue. The dead tissues are commonly invaded by a mixture of other organisms which may play a major role in putrefaction. (Anderson, 1976, pp. 170–171)

The bacteria usually grow in dead tissue, they cannot grow and multiply in living tissue because of oxygen. These are anaerobic bacteria.

Chapter thirty six: Bacteria are harmless   *139*

Oxygen interferes with growth and multiplication of these anaerobic bacteria. That's why bacteria growing in dead tissue are not harmful to living tissue.

> It has been learned that the intense oxidizing properties of high pressure oxygen (hyperbaric oxygen) can have valuable therapeutic effects in several important clinical conditions, probably the most successful use of hyperbaric oxygen has been in the treatment of gas gangrene. The bacteria that cause this condition, clostridial organisms, grow best under anaerobic conditions and stop growing at oxygen pressure greater than about 70 m.m. Hg ... Therefore, hyperbaric oxygenation of the tissues can frequently stop the infectious process entirely and this converts a condition that formerly was almost 100% (percent) fatal into one that is cured in most instance. (Raj, 2016, p. 410)

Whenever tissue oxygenation is less or blocked by some interference in blood supply, these saprophytic microorganisms grow in the body and produce disease.

> The most important prerequisite for the conversion of clostridial contamination of a wound to a progressive infection is an environment with low oxidation reduction potential, which permits spore germination and anaerobic growth. Local oxidation reduction potential can be reduced by failure of the blood supply to a contaminated area or by multiplication of other bacteria in the wound. Once multiplication and toxin production are established rapid invasion and destruction of healthy tissue follows. (Sande & Hook, 1983, p. 1009)

Now it is clear why bacteria from dead bodies cannot produce disease in healthy tissue, but when tissue oxygenation is reduced, these saprophytic microorganisms become dangerous to the body. Now again we can write that the concept of Kent is wrong regarding bacteria and disease. There is no necessity of giving an explanation of all examples that had been used by Hahnemann. Explanation of a few examples is sufficient.

I am giving one more example. Hahnemann saw "The slightest breath of air emitting from the body of a person affected with smallpox will suffice to produce this horrible disease in a healthy child" (Hahnemann, 1921/1993, p. 45). Then Hahnemann said, "Who can prove that some material portion of this substance has penetrated into our fluids or been absorbed" (Hahnemann, 1921/1993, p. 45). In this example, Hahnemann did not know that smallpox is due to a virus that can spread by air inhalation. "Direct transmission for short distances occurs through projection of droplets or droplet nuclei from the upper respiratory tract of an infected host" (Henderson, 1973, p. 107). Hahnemann did not know that viruses can transmit via respiratory route, that's why he was not able to understand how disease material can penetrate into the body and cause diseases. So, he never accepted external material as a disease agent. Hahnemann and Kent could not understand the reality and framed false homeopathic rules.

Microorganisms are not the only etiology for diseases. There are various diseases in which microorganism are never responsible. Genetics and internal factors are also responsible for many diseases. Hypertension, cardiac problems, carcinomas, diabetes, endocrinological abnormalities, arthritis, immunological diseases, schizophrenia, and mania are various examples where external material substance is not entered into the body.

References

Anderson, J. R. (1976). Type of infection. In J.R. Anderson (Ed.), *Muir's textbook of pathology* (10th ed., pp. 161–190). London, United Kingdom: ELBS & Edward Arnold.

Bison, A. L. (1983). Streptococcal infections. In R. G. Petersdorf, R. D. Adams, E. Braunwald, K. J. Isselbacher, J. B. Martin, & J. D. Wilson (Eds.), *Harrison's principle of internal medicine* (10th ed., pp. 929–935). New Delhi, India: McGraw Hill.

Corey, L. (1983). Rabies and other rhabdoviruses. In R. G. Petersdorf, R. D. Adams, E. Braunwald, K. J. Isselbacher, J. B. Martin, & J. D. Wilson (Eds.), *Harrison's principle of internal medicine* (10th ed., pp. 1136–1141). New Delhi, India: McGraw Hill.

Hahnemann, S. (1993). *Organon of medicine* (6th ed.). (W. Boericke, Trans.). New Delhi, India: B. Jain Publishers. (Original work published in 1921).

Hahnemann, S. (2017). *Organon of medicine* (6th ed.) (W. Boericke, Trans). New Delhi, India: B. Jain Publishers. (Original work published in 1921).

Henderson, D. A. (1973). Smallpox. In P. E. Sartwell, & E. Sartwell (Eds.), *Maxcy-Rosenau-preventive medicine and public health* (10th ed., pp. 105–116). New York, NY: Appleton-Century-Crofts (A publishing division of Prentice Hall).

Kent, J. T. (1993). *Lectures on homeopathic philosophy*. Delhi, India: B. Jain Publishers.

Modi, N. J. (1975). *Textbook of medical jurisprudence and toxicology* (Indian 9th ed.). Bombay, India: N.M. Tripathi, Publisher.

Chapter thirty six: Bacteria are harmless   *141*

Park, K. (1997). *Park's textbook of preventive and social medicine* (Indian 15th ed.). Jabalpur, India: Banarsidas Bhanot Publisher.

Raj, T. (2016). Applied respiratory physiology. In J. E. Hall, M. Viz, A. Kurpad, & T. Raj (Eds.), *Guyton and Hall textbook of medical physiology* (Second South Asia ed., pp. 405–411). Delhi, India: Elsevier (RELX India Pvt. Ltd).

Sande, M. A., & Hook, E. W. (1983). Other clostridial infections. In R. G. Petersdorf, R. D. Adams, E. Braunwald, K. J. Isselbacher, J. B. Martin, & J. D. Wilson (Eds.), *Harrison's principle of internal medicine* (10th ed., pp. 1009–1013). New Delhi, India: McGraw Hill.

chapter thirty seven

Hahnemann opposed old school of medicine

Basic concept of homeopathy – thirty seven

Hahnemann criticized derivation, imitation, and counterirritation by saying that they are unhelpful, injurious, and indirect modes of treatment. He also opposed large doses that were being used by old allopaths.

Argument

It has been observed by Hahnemann,

> The degenerated substances and impurities that appear in diseases are undeniably nothing more than products of disease, if abnormally deranged. Organisms which are expelled by the lather often violently enough ... Nature assists the diseased organism, resolves fever by perspiration, other diseases by vomiting, diarrhoea and bleeding from the anus, articular pains by suppurating ulcers of legs. (Hahnemann, 1921/1993, p. 51)

Hahnemann also said,

> Old school of medicine thought the best thing to do was to imitate nature, by means of stronger heterogeneous irritants applied to organs remote from the seat of disease and totally dissimilar to the affected tissues, they produce evacuations and generally kept then up in order to draw as it were the disease thither. In this imitation ... They endeavored to excite by force new symptoms in the tissues that are least diseased. (Hahnemann, 1921/1993, p. 52)

> To assist this derivative method, the old school of medicine employed the allied treatment by counter irritants, woollen garments to the bare skin,

DOI: 10.1201/9781003228622-37

144   *Homeopathy*

> foot baths, nauseant, … Substances to cause pain, inflammation and suppuration in near or distant parts as the application of horseradish, mustard plasters, cantharides, blisters, mezereum setons, issues, tartar emetic, ointments, moxa, actual cautery, acupuncture etc. by exciting pain in distant parts of body or by metastases and abscess by eruptions and suppurating ulcers. (Hahnemann, 1921/1993, p. 53)

Hahnemann rightly criticized this mode of treatment. I have said many times, Hahnemann opposed the old school of medicine, not the present advanced medical science. Hahnemann opposed derivation, imitation, and counterirritation by saying,

> It is an unhelpful and injurious indirect mode of treatment. The derivatives as well as the counter-irritant that led them to this inefficacious debilitating and hurtful practice of apparently ameliorating disease for a short time or removing them in such a manner that another and a worse disease was roused up to occupy the place of the first. Such a destructive plan cannot certainly be termed curing. (Hahnemann, 1921/1993, p. 54)

Hahnemann opposed the old school of medicine due to some other reasons also. He said that old allopaths had been using drugs in very large doses. Cinchona bark was being used for all epidemic intermittent fever with enormous doses. Condition of patient became worse than he was having during the fever. Similarly, due to large doses of Digitalis purpurea, patients had serious toxic effects, and death was very common (Hahnemann, 1921/1993, pp. 71–73).

Hahnemann criticized the old school of medicine by saying that the real action of prescribing medicinal substances was unknown. These drugs were non-beneficial, injurious to patients, torture them, waste their strength and fluids, and shorten their lives (Hahnemann, 1921/1993, pp. 75–79).

Conclusively, it can be said that Hahnemann's criticism of the old school of medicine or old allopathy was correct. The concept and methodology of the old school of medicine can never be correlated with the modern advanced medical science. The old school of medicine was not accurate. Today we are able to say with certainty that homeopathy is also wrong.

Reference

Hahnemann, S. (1993). *Organon of medicine* (6th ed.) (W. Boericke, Trans.). New Delhi, India: B. Jain Publishers. (Original work published in 1921).

chapter thirty eight

Termination of acute and chronic disease

Basic concept of homeopathy – thirty eight

It is only the slighter and acute disease that tends to terminate quietly in resolution or death. All chronic diseases of mankind cannot be cured spontaneously. They increase even more over the years. They never pass away from themselves but increase and are aggravated even till death. There are three chronic diseases: (a) syphilis, (b) sycosis, and (c) psora.

Argument

Now it is being analyzed here, how Hahnemann, Kent, and their followers made mistakes. The most important part of discovery of therapeutics is knowledge of normal course and normal process of disease when external therapeutic measures are not provided. Without knowing the normal course of disease, it is totally useless to claim successful treatment of disease.

All diseases are not always fatal. Today AIDS is a fatal disease. Once a person is infected with AIDS virus, he will definitely die. Nothing can save him. Many diseases have spontaneous cure. Tropical diseases are usually resolved spontaneously. Tropical diseases mean diseases that originated due to external infective agents and transmitted by usually dirty water, dirty food, and unhygienic surroundings.

By treatment, the course of disease is shortened, intensity of symptomatology is reduced, and morbidity and mortality are also lessened. But to know the importance of treatment, a comparative study with control is a must. Without doing comparative and therapeutic trials, we cannot establish the utility of a treatment. If a disease is going to be resolved spontaneously and somebody says, "This cure is due to my treatment", then it is not an accurate comment. The same mistakes were made by Hahnemann, Kent, and their followers. They did not study the normal course of the diseases and blindly claimed that they had been able to cure many chronic diseases with their homeopathic remedies.

Hahnemann divided disease into two groups. "The diseases to which man is liable are either rapid morbid processes of the abnormally

DOI: 10.1201/9781003228622-38

145

146   *Homeopathy*

deranged vital force, which have a tendency to finish their course more or less quickly, but always in a moderate time these are termed acute disease" (Hahnemann, 1921/1993, p. 159).

Hahnemann further writes,

> It is only the slighter and acute diseases that tend when the natural period of their course has expired, to terminate quietly in resolution as it is called with or without the employment of not very aggressive allopathic remedies, vital force having regained its power, then gradually substitutes the normal condition for the derangement of the health that has now ceased to exist. (Hahnemann, 1921/1993, p. 52)

Hahnemann also writes,

> Allied to these (acute disease) are those diseases in which many persons are attacked with very similar sufferings from the same cause (epidemically); these diseases generally become infectious (contagious) when they prevail among thickly congregated masses of human beings. Thence arise fevers in each instance of a peculiar nature and because the cases of disease have an identical origin, they set up in all those they affect an identical morbid process which when left to itself terminates in a moderate period of time in death or recovery. (Hahnemann, 1921/1993, p. 160)

Now it is clear by the above statement that Hahnemann was of the opinion that some acute diseases are resolved spontaneously without any external treatment.

Hahnemann again raised questions against the old school of medicine.

> It remains a very doubtful question whether the natural process of recovery in acute diseases is really at all shortened or facilitated by this interference of the old school, as the latter cannot act otherwise than the vital force, namely indirectly, but its derivative and counter-irritant treatment is much more injurious and much more debilitating. (Hahnemann, 1921/1993, p. 69)

Chapter thirty eight: Termination of acute and chronic disease 147

The objection of Hahnemann was right against the old school of medicine because no controlled study was done and a normal course of the disease was also not known to the old school of medicine. The same questions can also be raised against homeopathy when the treatment of chronic diseases is concerned. Hahnemann knew this fact that some acute diseases are resolved spontaneously without any treatment. For this, Hahnemann should be appreciated. When the question of chronic diseases arises, Hahnemann was also wrong.

Hahnemann writes regarding chronic diseases,

> They are diseases of such a character that with small often imperceptible beginnings, dynamically derange the living organism, each in its peculiar manner, and cause it gradually to deviate from the healthy condition in such a way that the automatic life energy called vital force, whose office is to preserve the health only opposes to them at the commencement and during their process imperfect unsuitable, useless resistance but is unable of itself to extinguished them but helplessly suffer itself to be ever more and more abnormally deranged until at length the organism is destroyed, these are termed chronic diseases. (Hahnemann, 1921/1993, p. 159)

Hahnemann also writes,

> All chronic diseases of mankind, even those left to themselves ... They evermore increase with the years and during the whole of man's lifetime and they cannot be diminished by the strength belonging even to the most robust constitution ... They never pass away from themselves but increase and are aggravated even till death ... first syphilis which I have also called the general chancre disease, then sycosis or fig wart disease and finally the chronic disease which lies at the foundation of the eruption of itch psora ... psora is the oldest miasmatic chronic disease known to us. Just as tedious as syphilis and sycosis and, therefore, not to be extinguished before the last breath of the longest human life, unless it is thoroughly cured, since not even the most robust constitution is able to destroy and extinguish it by its own proper strength. (Hahnemann, 1835/1990, p. 9)

It was also said by Hahnemann, "In severe acute and chronic diseases which constitute by far the greatest portion of all human ailments, crude nature and the old school are equally powerless" (Hahnemann, 1921/1993, p. 52).

In these paragraphs, Hahnemann wanted to say that chronic diseases are not able to resolve spontaneously. For the treatment of chronic diseases, drugs have to be given. Hahnemann treated chronic diseases with drugs and he got the results. He thought that he was curing the disease by using drugs. But in fact the chronic diseases, treated by Hahnemann, were resolved spontaneously. He did not know this fact. He thought erroneously that his drugs were effective in treating chronic diseases and he wrongly formulated the law of homeopathy.

Hahnemann had the misconception that

> True natural chronic diseases are those that arise from a chronic miasm always going on increasing and growing worse, notwithstanding the best mental and corporeal regimen and torment the patient to the end of his life with ever aggravated suffering. These, excepting those produced by medical malpractice, are the most numerous and greatest scourges of the human race; for the most robust constitution, the best regulated mode of living and the most vigorous energy of the vital force are insufficient for their eradication. (Hahnemann, 1921/1993, p. 166)

References

Hahnemann, S. (1990). *The chronic diseases-their peculiar nature and their homeopathic cure* (L. Tafel, Trans.). New Delhi, India: B. Jain Publishers. (Original work published in 1835).

Hahnemann, S. (1993). *Organon of medicine* (6th ed.) (W. Boericke, Trans.). New Delhi, India: B. Jain Publishers. (Original work published in 1921).

chapter thirty nine

Syphilis causes termination of life

Basic concept of homeopathy – thirty nine

Syphilis alone is to some extent known as such a chronic miasmatic disease, which when uncured ceases only with the termination of life.

Argument

Hahnemann mentioned the three causes of diseases: psora, syphilis, and sycosis. Causes of acute diseases are "Transient explosion of latent psora which spontaneously returns to its dormant state, if the acute disease were not of too violent a character and were soon quelled" (Hahnemann, 1921/1993, p. 160).

According to Homeopaths, causes of chronic disease are psora, syphilis, and sycosis. This syphilis mainly confused Hahnemann, Kent, and their followers. Syphilis is one of the main diseases, which is responsible for the development of homeopathy. Hahnemann writes, "Syphilis alone has been to some extent known as such a chronic miasmatic disease, which when uncured ceases only with the termination of life" (Hahnemann, 1921/1993, p. 166).

Hahnemann did not know actual etiology, pathogenesis, and prognosis of syphilis, and other sexually transmitted diseases. There are five main sexually transmitted diseases: gonorrheas, syphilis, chancroid, lymphogranuloma venereum, and granuloma inguinale. There are also other diseases having bacterial viral, protozoal, and fungal etiology that might be considered sexually transmitted diseases, with 23 sexually transmitting pathogens. Diagnosis and detection of specific etiological agents by microscope and serological testing are very much important, otherwise diagnosis is very difficult. Hahnemann did not accept external microorganism as etiology, that's why at the time of Hahnemann, it was not possible to diagnose specific sexually transmitted disease. As mentioned in history of medicine,

> The erroneous concept that gonorrhea, chancroid and syphilis were the same disease was strengthened by John Hunter, who developed syphilis following self inoculation with gonorrhoea pus in 1767.

DOI: 10.1201/9781003228622-39

149

> These three diseases were finally distinguished in the mid-1800s, although their aetiologies were not established until the turn of this century. Gummas were not recognized as being syphilitic in origin until this century. The discovery of Treponema pallidum in serum from secondary lesions was made by Schaudinn in 1905 and was confirmed by Landsteiner in 1906. Wasserman introduced the complete fixation test for the diagnosis of syphilis in the same year. (Holmes, 1983, p. 1035)

And this information should be kept in mind by readers that Hahnemann did his work during 1800–1830.

Now we are concentrating on the comparative analytical study of syphilis. We will compare the information regarding syphilis, which were present at the time of Hahnemann and what we have today.

I have written previously that Hahnemann presumed syphilis cannot be resolved spontaneously. Homeopathic drugs have to be given for the treatment of syphilis. But today by normal observations of syphilitic patients without giving any treatment, we have found that many patients were cured spontaneously. Little knowledge of syphilis is necessary to understand facts of homeopathy.

Syphilis is a chronic infection due to *Treponema pallidum*. It is systemic from the beginning, runs a chronic course characterized by florid features at times but by long periods of latency at other times. The subdivision between early and late syphilis is two years. It may be latent throughout and its course is variable. After an incubation period of 9–90 days, the primary lesion or chancre develops at the site of infection usually on the genitalia. A small pink macule appears, which becomes papular and ulcerated. The primary chancre heals, and six to eight weeks later, malaise, headache, and fever appear. Four signs appear – a rash, lymphadenopathy, condylomata, and mucous patches – though any of them may be absent. Condyloma lata is a large flat papule that develops around the anus, rarely eye, joints, bone, or abdominal viscera; the nervous system may be affected. After several months, the secondary changes gradually disappear to be followed by a latent period (Griffin et al, 1999, pp. 184–187).

Latency may persist for many years. Tertiary stage takes ten or more years to develop and affects skin, mucous membrane, subcutaneous tissue, submucosa, and long bone mainly. The characteristic finding is called gumma. Lesions run a long benign course. In the quaternary stage, there are two main conditions: one is cardiovascular syphilis and the second is neurosyphilis. These usually take longer to develop morbidity and may lead to the patient's death. These stages develop after 15–20 years of primary infection.

Chapter thirty nine: Syphilis causes termination of life   151

Now we should know the normal prognosis of syphilitic patients when treatment is not being given. Medical observations say,

> Following the secondary stage, untreated adults fall into four groups (a) One-third remain symptomless throughout life with a persistent positive W.R. (Wassermann reaction – an antigen antibody reaction), (b) One-third are likewise symptomless, with a W.R. which ultimately becomes negative, (c) One-sixth develop early tertiary symptoms which abort spontaneously, (d) One-sixth develop and suffer from disease affecting many different systems of the body. The first two groups are termed latent syphilis. It is not possible to know beforehand whether the disease will remain latent or whether it will cause future complications in some vital part. (Warner, 1964, p. 729)

In another study, it has been found,

> The primary lesion appears at the site of inoculation and persists for 2 to 6 weeks and then heals spontaneously ... Some patients enter the latent stage without ever developing secondary lesions ... The secondary lesions subside within 2 to 6 weeks and the patient enters the latent stage, which is detectable only by serological testing ... About one third of patients with untreated latent syphilis develop clinically apparent tertiary disease. (Holmes, 1983, pp. 1035–1036)

"Oslo study and Tuskegee study show that about one-third of patients with untreated syphilis develop clinical or pathological evidence of tertiary syphilis, about one-fourth die as a direct result of tertiary syphilis" (Holmes, 1983, p. 1037).

By analyzing the results of normal prognosis of syphilitic patients, it can be concluded that 60–70% of syphilitic patients are cured spontaneously without giving any treatment. The another important aspect of syphilis is "The average interval from infection to onset of symptoms is 5 to 10 years for meningovascular syphilis, 20 years for general paresis and 25 to 30 years for tabes dorsalis" (Holmes, 1983, p. 1038).

Twenty to thirty percent of syphilitic patients develop neurological or cardiovascular complications. But development of these complications

152 *Homeopathy*

takes a long time of 5–30 years. Observation of patients up to 30 years would not have been possible at the time of Hahnemann and Kent. Sixty to seventy percent of syphilitic patients are cured spontaneously and the remaining patients take a very long time to develop complications. After short-time observations, it can be concluded wrongly that all syphilitic patients have been cured by any treatment that has been given to such patients. Hahnemann and Kent made these mistakes and they provided useless homeopathic treatment to syphilitic patients and concluded wrongly that they had cured syphilis.

Hahnemann writes,

> The chancre appears after an impure coition usually between the seventh and fourteenth days, first as a little pustule which changes into an impure ulcer with raised borders and stinging pains which if not cured remains standing on the same place during man's lifetime, only increasing with years while the secondary symptoms of the venereal disease, syphilis cannot break out as long as it exists. (Hahnemann, 1835/1990, p. 87)

Hahnemann agreed with this statement that syphilis always follows the destruction of the chancre by local application. Hahnemann also writes, "I have never in my practice of more than fifty years seen any trace of venereal disease break out, so long as the chancre remained untouched in its place even if this were a space of several years for it never passes away of itself and even it had largely increased its place" (Hahnemann, 1835/1990, p. 89).

Today we know about syphilis that primary chancre heals spontaneously, and six to eight weeks later, secondary symptoms appear irrespective of external manipulation of chancre. Systemic manifestations of syphilis are not related to destruction or some sort of external treatment of chancre. If chancre remains for prolonged time, then definitely it is not syphilis; it is something else. In my opinion, Hahnemann was not able to differentiate between chancre and chancroid. He wrongly labeled chancroid and told them chancre. Actually they were chancroid not chancre.

Haemophilus ducreyi is a bacterium caused chancroid.

> Chancroid or soft chancre is a sexually transmitted infection, characterized by painful genital ulceration ... The incidence of chancroid is unknown owing to inaccurate clinical diagnosis and incomplete reporting ... Chancroid is more common than

Chapter thirty nine: Syphilis causes termination of life 153

> syphilis ... In contrast to syphilis the chancroidal
> ulcer in males is painful and not indurated ... Acute,
> painful tender inflammatory inguinal adenopa-
> thy occurs in almost 50 percent of patients and fre-
> quently unilateral. If the patient is untreated, the
> involved nodes become matted forming a unilocular
> suppurative bubo. The overlying skin becomes ery-
> thematous and tense and finally ruptures forming a
> deep single ulcer ... The chancre of primary syphilis
> is indurated and the associated adenopathy is bilat-
> eral, nontender and nonsuppurative ... Untreated
> chancroidal ulcers persist for long period of time
> and often progress. Small lesions may heal within
> 2 to 4 weeks. (Holmes & Ronald, 1983, pp. 973–974)

Chancroid rarely causes systemic symptoms.

Hahnemann described syphilitic chancre that "It has been substituted by a far more painful substitute, the bubo, which hastens onward to suppuration" (Hahnemann, 1835/1990, p. 88). This indicates clearly Hahnemann was confused. He was not able to differentiate between syphilitic chancre and chancroid. Chancroid is also a self-limiting disease.

> Chancroid (Soft chancre) is an acute, specific,
> localized self limiting autoinoculable infectious
> disease almost always acquired through sexual
> contact ... During medieval times chancroid was
> not distinguished from the initial lesion of syphilis.
> Gonorrhoea and Syphilis were differentiated about
> 1831, but it was not until 1850 that soft chancre was
> distinguished from the initial lesion of syphilis and
> later designated chancroid (chancre like) ... The
> ulcers of chancroid are painful and contain pus and
> may rupture spontaneously ... Most commonly the
> disease is self limiting but in some cases with rela-
> tively prolonged disability and tissue destruction
> may ensue. (Fleming, 1973, pp. 240–241)

References

Fleming, W. L. (1973). Venereal diseases. In P. E. Sartwell, & E. Sartwell (Eds.), *Maxcy-Rosenau-preventive medicine and public health* (10th ed., pp. 229–246). New York, NY: Appleton-Century-Crofts (A publishing division of Prentice Hall).

Griffin, G. E., Sissons, J. G. P., Chiodini, P. L., & Mitchell, D. M. (1999). Diseases due to infection. In C. Haslett, E. R. Chillers, J. A. A. Hunter, & N. A. Boon (Eds.), *Davidson's principles and practice of medicine* (18th ed., pp. 56–190). Edinburgh, United Kingdom: Churchill Livingstone.

Hahnemann, S. (1990). *The chronic diseases – their peculiar nature and their homeopathic cure* (L. Tafel, Trans.). New Delhi, India: B. Jain Publishers. (Original work published in 1835).

Hahnemann, S. (1993). *Organon of medicine* (6th ed.) (W. Boericke, Trans.). New Delhi, India: B. Jain Publishers. (Original work published in 1921).

Holmes, K. K. (1983). Syphilis. In R. G. Petersdorf, R. D. Adams, E. Braunwald, K. J. Isselbacher, J. B. Martin, & J. D. Wilson (Eds.), *Harrison's principle of internal medicine* (10th ed., pp. 1034–1045). New Delhi, India: McGraw Hill.

Holmes, K. K., & Ronald, A. R. (1983). Chancroid. In R. G. Petersdorf, R. D. Adams, E. Braunwald, K. J. Isselbacher, J. B. Martin, & J. D. Wilson (Eds.), *Harrison's principle of internal medicine* (10th ed., pp. 973–974). New Delhi, India: McGraw Hill.

Warner, E. C. (1964). *Savill's system of clinical medicine* (14th ed.). London, United Kingdom: Edward Arnold Publisher.

chapter forty

Treatment of syphilis

Basic concept of homeopathy – forty

Hahnemann writes regarding the treatment of syphilis. It needs only one little dose of the best mercurial remedy in order to cure thoroughly and forever the whole syphilis with its chancre within 14 days. He also used arsenic in the treatment of syphilis in a single dose.

Argument

"In the past potassium iodide, mercury, bismuth and organic arsenical compounds were used in syphilis. Mercury was originally used for syphilis but was superseded by bismuth and arsphenamine" (Warner, 1964, p. 731). These metallic compounds are highly toxic to the body; that's why they are not used nowadays. They have been replaced by antibiotics today.

> When mercury was being used in the treatment of syphilis by oral route, the medication had been administered several times a day for a long period of time … The proto iodide of mercury in doses of 1/5 to 1/2 grain was probably the most commonly administered salt. It is powerful, containing 61% of the metal but it is very liable to cause intestinal irritation and diarrhoea … Mercury with chalk in a dose of 1 to 3 grains or the tannate of mercury in 1/2 to 1 grain dose were appropriate forms of medication … Injection of soluble mercurial salts were also used for a long period of time. (Gottheil, 1913, pp. 361–435)

Regarding injectable mercurial compounds in the treatment of syphilis, it has been mentioned,

> In the first case a soluble mercurial salt is thrown almost directly into the blood giving an immediate most vigorous therapeutic effect but one which if that action is to be sustained requires repetition of

DOI: 10.1201/9781003228622-40

medication every day. Objective symptoms such as skin eruption and ulcerative lesion begin to improve in a day or two. It is the subjective symptoms however that show the therapeutic effect of injections most brilliantly. Improvement in general feeling begins in a few hours. Symptoms disappear and lesions heal with rapidity. The usual single parental dose of mercury compound was 0.065 gram. (Gottheil, 1913, pp. 361–435)

Mercury should be administered in compound form. Doses that were used by Hahnemann are as follows, Hahnemann writes,

In syphilis, it needs only one little dose of the best mercurial remedy in order to cure thoroughly and forever the whole syphilis with its chancre within fourteen days. I formerly used the billionth dynamization (ii) of this preparation, although the preparation of the higher potency (iv, vi, viii) and finally the decillionth potency show some advantages in their quick penetrating and yet mild action for this purpose, but in cases where a second or third dose (however seldom needed) should be found necessary a lower potency then be taken. (Hahnemann, 1828/1990, pp. 90–95)

Hahnemann himself writes regarding the potency of drugs. "The material part of the medicine is lessened with each degree of dynamization 50000 times … The thirtieth thus progressively prepared would give a fraction almost impossible to be expressed in numbers" (Hahnemann, 1921/1993, pp. 294–295). "The degree of dynamization is frequently so expressed that only the exponent showing how often one hundred has been multiplied into itself is expressed" (Hahnemann, 1835/1990, p. 150).

The above description shows that one decillionth dilution means 10^{60} dilution, which is equal to thirtieth potency. If one gram drug is dissolved into 10^{60} ml of water or alcohol, then it will be equal to thirtieth potency. We can say that such dilution will not contain any drug molecule. How can a drug of this dilution with only one dose cure a disease? On the other hand, mercury compounds in doses of 0.065 g, many times a day for prolonged periods, were being given for the treatment of syphilis. Therefore, we can say, homeopathic drugs mean no drug. It is just a placebo. The positive results claimed by homeopathic drugs are actually the result of the spontaneous cure.

Chapter forty: Treatment of syphilis 157

Hahnemann committed one more mistake. When external chancre remained localized and resolved spontaneously or remained localized without systemic manifestations, Hahnemann said it was syphilis that had been cured by antisyphilitic drug. Here, Hahnemann was wrong. It was actually a chancroid that usually never gives systemic manifestations, remains localized, or cures spontaneously.

If systemic manifestations of syphilis were present, Hahnemann thought, "He can cure these patients by antipsoric drug in addition to antisyphilitic drug". In view of Hahnemann, systemic manifestations of syphilis were due to psora. Here again, he was wrong. Actually systemic manifestations of the secondary stage of syphilis heal spontaneously. This healing was not due to antipsoric drugs advised by Hahnemann, but he thought wrongly. He writes, "Psora which had as yet been latent within him has been brought to its development and has broken out into chronic ailments and these irrepressibly combine with the internal syphilis" (Hahnemann, 1835/1990, p. 93).

Regarding false belief of curing syphilis, Masters and Johnson write clearly,

> The chancre generally appears two to four weeks after infection, ... chancre is painless in 75 percent of cases ... The chancre usually heals within four to six weeks, leading to the erroneous belief that the problem went away. Secondary syphilis begins anywhere from one week to six months after the chancre heals if effective treatment was not received ... Because of the diversity of symptoms syphilis is sometimes called the great imitator. The symptoms of the secondary stage of syphilis usually last three to six months but can come and go periodically. After all, symptoms disappear ... Fifty to 70 percent of people with untreated syphilis stay in this stage for the rest of their lives. Remainder passes on to the tertiary stage or late syphilis which involves serious heart problems, eye problems, brain and spinal cord damage. These complications cause blindness, paralysis, death. (Masters et al., 1986, pp. 534–535)

Such developments may take up to 20–30 years.

For such a prolonged period, it could not have been possible to observe patients to know the fate of homeopathic treatment, so Hahnemann wrongly concluded that he had cured syphilitic patients

158 *Homeopathy*

by homeopathy. The same mistake was made by Kent. Kent writes, "Homeopathic treatment strikes at the root of the evil … that the chancre that is painful will become painless … Suppressed manifestations must come back and they will come back under appropriate treatment" (Kent, 1993, pp. 142–143).

Chancres of syphilis are painless already. There is no question of homeopathic treatment that can make syphilitic chancre painless. It was a wrong observation of Kent. Kent writes suppressed manifestations must come back under treatment. It was also the wrong comment of Kent. Normally the first stage of syphilis is spontaneously suppressed. Then, after some time, a secondary stage appears, which is also suppressed spontaneously, and after a gap of years, a third stage appears. "The symptoms of the secondary stage of syphilis usually last 3 to six months but can come and go periodically" (Masters et al., 1986, p. 535).

This periodicity of appearance and disappearance of symptomatology of syphilis gave the wrong impression to Kent that reappearance of symptomatology of syphilis was due to homeopathic treatment. But it was not the fact. Periodicity of symptomatology in syphilis, and in 70–80% of patients, the total disappearance of symptoms after the second stage without any treatment is the normal course of syphilis. From the above discussion, we can say that the comment of Kent, "Suppressed manifestations must come back under appropriate treatment" is wrong.

Regarding the frequency of doses, Hahnemann writes, "A single one of which sufficiently attenuated and potentized, would have sufficed to cure all the disease in the whole habitable world for which this drug is the suitable remedy" (Hahnemann, 1835/1990, pp. 322). I am giving an example of arsenicum album. Regarding dose of arsenic, Hahnemann says, "Homeopathy which by unwearied, multiplied experiments discovered that it is only rare cases that more than a decillionth of a grain of arsenic should be given" (Hahnemann, 1835/1990, pp. 322). One decillionth dilution means $1:10^{60}$ dilution. Hahnemann, Kent, and we all agree that in such dilutions, it is very difficult to find a single molecule of a drug. Example of syphilis is being given, where the causative organism of syphilis is *Treponema pallidum*. How can *T. pallidum* be killed by a drug that contains not even a single molecule of drug?

Hahnemann said that the best homeopathic drug should be given in a single dose only with 10^{60} dilution. How can a drug kill *T. pallidum* or other organisms in a single dose with 10^{60} dilution? Hahnemann used arsenic for the treatment of syphilis in a single dose. How arsenic in one globule that contains only 0.5 ml of arsenic with 10^{60} dilution can be effective in the treatment of syphilis.

Chapter forty: Treatment of syphilis 159

To understand the importance of dose in treatment, an example of penicillin must be learnt. Penicillin is the drug of choice in the treatment of syphilis and it is highly effective in treponema.

> To be effective in syphilis and other treponematoses, high blood concentration of penicillin 0.03 units per ml. must be attained. Moreover because penicillin only attacks actively dividing organisms and treponemas divide only slowly, this high concentration must be maintained for periods upto 15 days to ensure that all the organisms have been killed and to prevent relapses. In syphilis, penicillin is best given in daily intramuscular doses of 600000 to one million units of procaine penicillin G. (Crossland, 1980, pp. 861–862)

Neoarsphenamine, an arsenic compound, had been used in syphilis previously. "Neoarsphenamine 0.6 g is made into solution with sterile distilled water 6 ml and the freshly made solution is injected intravenously once a week for 10 weeks" (Warner, 1964, p. 732).

Arsenic compounds are not used today due to toxicity. But if we use arsenic, then required doses have to be administered in the treatment of syphilis to kill *T. pallidum*. The dilutions of arsenic used by Hahnemann cannot kill the syphilitic microorganism. When homeopathy does not accept *T. pallidum* as a causative organism of syphilis, then the question of killing treponema cannot be raised in homeopathy. This truth should be accepted by homeopaths that the causative organism of syphilis is *T. pallidum*, because in the absence of treponema, syphilis cannot be produced in human beings.

Now conclusively we can say, in syphilis, after secondary stage, it is more or less impossible to say on the basis of healed symptoms only that disease has been cured by drug or it has been cured spontaneously or disease is in remission phase because this disease may remain symptomless up to 20–30 years. Observation up to 20–30 years, after disappearance of symptom of second or tertiary stage of syphilis, is required to know that disease has been cured spontaneously or diseased state is present. Development of neurosyphilis, cardiovascular syphilis, or other symptoms, which develop only after prolonged interval, are only symptomatological evidence of late syphilis. After secondary stage, syphilis may remain silent for years. It is very difficult to say which patient will develop late syphilis and which patient will get cured spontaneously. As we know, only 17–20% of syphilitic patients develop late symptoms of syphilis, remaining patients are cured spontaneously.

Hahnemann did not know about the normal course of syphilis. So he made a wrong judgment regarding its cure. He wrongly presumed that he had been able to cure syphilis by homeopathic medicine. Then he made an erroneous concept of homeopathy.

As we know, the average interval from infection to onset of symptoms is 5–10 years for meningovascular syphilis, 20 years for tabes dorsalis. These varieties of syphilis that develop after prolonged intervals usually do not have skin lesions. These varieties of syphilis develop after remission of the secondary stage of syphilis. Without a serological test, it is very difficult to tell that these varieties are sequelae of primary syphilis or independent of syphilis. At the time of Hahnemann, serological test of syphilis was not available; that's why he was not able to detect syphilis in those patients who have neurological or cardiovascular complications. "Even in 1875, William Welch's report that syphilis was a cause of aortic aneurysm was ignored, until 30 years later, Reuter demonstrated spirochetes within the vessel walls in active aortitis" (Lowy & Androphy, 1993, p. 2619).

Thus, Hahnemann must have wrongly interpreted the cure of syphilitic patients and developed the wrong concept regarding the treatment of syphilis. Misinterpretation of the treatment of syphilis is the most important cause in the development of homeopathy.

In the description of syphilis, Kent writes, "Dissimilar repel each other and similars attract and cure each other" (Kent, 1993, p. 141). But what is the fact, "Untreated syphilis may make people more susceptible to other diseases or individuals who get syphilis coincidentally may be more susceptible to other diseases" (Holmes, 1983, p. 103). Kent also writes in the homeopathic treatment of syphilis, "Bubo will be hastened to suppuration when it would not otherwise suppurate" (Kent, 1993, p. 142). But the fact is "The chancre of primary syphilis is indurated and the associated adenopathy is bilateral, nontender and non suppurative" (Holmes & Ronald, 1983, p. 974).

In this way, we can conclude that these people of homeopathy did not have proper knowledge of diseases; that's why they erroneously diagnosed the disease. They were not able to differentiate one disease from another due to a lack of knowledge.

References

Crossland, J. (1980). *Lewis's pharmacology* (5th ed.). New York, NY: Churchill Livingston.

Gottheil, E. S. (1913). The general & special treatment of syphilis. In F. Forchheimer (Ed.), *Therapeutics of internal diseases* (Vol 2, pp. 361–437). Sydney, Australia: Butterworth & Co.

Chapter forty: Treatment of syphilis 161

Hahnemann, S. (1990). *The chronic diseases – Their peculiar nature and their homeo-pathic cure* (L. Tafel, Trans.). New Delhi, India: B. Jain Publishers. (Original work published in 1835).

Hahnemann, S. (1993). *Organon of medicine* (6th ed.) (W. Boericke, Trans.). New Delhi, India: B. Jain Publishers (P) Ltd. (Original work published in 1921).

Holmes, K. K., & Ronald, A. R. (1983). Chancroid. In R. G. Petersdorf, R. D. Adams, E. Braunwald, K. J. Isselbacher, J. B. Martin, & J. D. Wilson (Eds.), *Harrison's principle of internal medicine* (10th ed., pp. 973–974). New Delhi, India: McGraw Hill.

Holmes, K. K. (1983). Syphilis. In R. G. Petersdorf, R. D. Adams, E. Braunwald, K. J. Isselbacher, J. B. Martin, & J. D. Wilson (Eds.), *Harrison's principle of internal medicine* (10th ed., pp. 1034–1045). New Delhi, India: McGraw Hill.

Kent, J. T. (1993). *Lectures on homeopathic philosophy*. Delhi, India: B. Jain Publishers.

Lowy, D. R., & Androphy, E. J. (1993). Warts. In T. B. Fitzpatrick, A. Z. Eisen, K. Wolff, I. M. Freedberg, & K. F. Austen (Eds.), *Dermatology in general medicine* (4th ed., Vol. 2, pp. 2611–2620). New York, NY: McGraw Hill.

Masters, W. H., Johnson, V. E., & Kolodny, R. C. (1986). *Masters & Johnson on sex and human loving*. Mumbai, India: Jaico Publishing House.

Warner, E. C. (Ed.). (1964). *Savill's system of clinical medicine* (14th ed.). London, United Kingdom: Edward Arnold Publisher.

chapter forty one

Sycosis

Basic concept of homeopathy – forty one

Homeopathy says, sycosis, the condylomatous disease, is ineradicable by the vital force without proper medicinal treatment. Sycosis is revealed by cauliflower-like growth. When discharge of gonorrhea is suppressed by allopathic injection, sycosis is established in the body.

Argument

We have discussed syphilis in detail and reached a conclusion that Hahnemann and Kent were wrong and they made wrong impressions about the treatment of syphilis. Now we shall discuss sycosis, second chronic miasm, and we will be able to prove that Hahnemann was again wrong in the study of sycosis.

Hahnemann writes (1999),

> According to all investigations, only three chronic miasms are found, the diseases caused by which manifest themselves through local symptoms and from which most, if not all, the chronic diseases originate; namely first syphilis which I have also called the venereal chancre disease, then sycosis or the fig wart disease and finally the chronic disease which lies at foundation of the eruption of itch i.e. the psora. (Hahnemann, 1999, pp. 34–35)

"All chronic diseases of mankind ... never pass away of themselves but increase and are aggravated even till death" (Hahnemann, 1999, p. 34).

Syphilis and sycosis were called two venereal diseases (Hahnemann, 1999, p. 33). Hahnemann also writes,

> Syphilis and sycosis both have an advantage over the itch disease in this that the chancre or bubo in the one and fig wart in the other never leave the external parts until they have been either mischievously destroyed through external repressive remedies or have been in a rational manner removed through

DOI: 10.1201/9781003228622-41

the simultaneous internal cure of the whole disease. The venereal disease cannot therefore break out so long as the chancre is not artificially destroyed by external applications, nor can the secondary ailments of sycosis break out so long as the big wart has not been destroyed by faulty practice, for these local symptoms which act as substitute for the internal disease, remain standing even until the end of man's life and prevent the breaking out of internal disease. (Hahnemann, 1999, p. 40)

Hahnemann writes regarding the treatment of syphilis and sycosis,

It is therefore just as easy to heal them even in their whole extent i.e. thoroughly through their specific internal medicines which need only to be continued until these local symptoms (chancre and fig wart) which are in their nature unchangeable except through artificial external applications are thoroughly healed. Then we may be quite certain that we have thoroughly cured the internal disease i.e., syphilis and sycosis. (Hahnemann, 1999, p. 40)

Hahnemann writes in the organon of medicine, "Sycosis is the condylomatous disease equally ineradicable by the vital force without proper medicinal treatment ... Sycosis is revealed by cauliflower-like growth" (Hahnemann, 1921/1993, pp. 166–167).

Some homeopaths explained, any type of muscular growth, which is abnormal, is actually sycosis. Sometimes warts like cauliflower or like a bunch of grapes appear also due to sycosis. External piles are also labeled due to sycosis (Ghatak, 1931/1938, pp. 241–242).

It is mentioned in homeopathy that gonorrhea is due to sexual relation with diseased females, and when discharge of gonorrhea is suppressed by injections of allopathic doctors, sycosis is established in the body (Ghatak, 1931/1938, pp. 59–60).

References

Ghatak, N. (1938). *Cause and cure of chronic diseases* (4th ed.) (C. S. Pathak, Trans.). Kolkata, India: Dr. S.M. Bhattacharya. (Original work published in 1931).

Hahnemann, S. (1993). *Organon of medicine* (6th ed.) (W. Boericke, Trans.). New Delhi, India: B. Jain Publishers (P) Ltd. (Original work published in 1921).

Hahnemann, S. (1999). *The chronic diseases (theoretical part)* (Reprint ed.). New Delhi, India: B Jain Publishers.

chapter forty two

Venereal diseases

Basic concept of homeopathy – forty two

Hahnemann included all venereal diseases into two groups: one where lesion is ulcerative or papular labeled as syphilitic miasm and second where lesion is like external growth or discharge from urethra labeled as sycosis. Both were called two venereal diseases that were treated with the mercury, thuja, and nitric acid by Hahnemann.

Argument

Today we know that there are five common venereal diseases also known as sexually transmitted diseases. These are syphilis, gonorrhea, chancroid, lymphogranuloma venereum, and granuloma inguinale. One more which we shall include in our discussion is genital wart or condyloma acuminata. And the next genital herpes is important for the analytical aspect of homeopathy. We shall discuss these seven diseases because these all spread by coitus.

To differentiate these all diseases from each other is not easy by only clinical inspection. "Early donovanosis (granuloma inguinale) may be mistaken for the primary chancre or condyloma latum of syphilis ... Chronic ulcerative or cicatricial changes may resemble lymphogranuloma venereum. Amoebiasis can produce penile lesions resembling donovanosis (Granuloma inguinale)" (Holmes, 1983b, pp. 1000–1001).

Isolation of infective agents which may be bacteria, virus, chlamydia, or other agents and serological tests are only two confirmatory processes to make a definite diagnosis. Both these methods were not present at the time of Hahnemann. Hahnemann and his followers must not have been able to make an accurate diagnosis. They were confused and not able to differentiate one disease from another.

Second most important aspect is regarding treatment. Hahnemann thought, these all above mentioned sexually transmitted diseases are due to chronic miasm and cannot be cured spontaneously. But the fact is that the dilutions used by Hahnemann had no drug. Such homeopathic drugs are actually no drug. Homeopathy treatment is actually no treatment.

DOI: 10.1201/9781003228622-42

Hahnemann writes,

> These excrescences usually first manifest themselves on the genitals and appears usually but not with a sort of gonorrhea from the urethra, several days or several weeks even many weeks after infection through coition, more rarely they appear dry, and like warts more frequently soft and spongy, emitting a specifically fetid fluid ... bleeding easily and in the form of a coxcomb or a cauliflower ... Usually in gonorrhea of this kind the discharge is from the beginning thickish like pus ... the body of penis swollen somewhat hard and in some cases covered on the back with glandular tubercles, and very painful to touch. (Hahnemann, 1999, pp. 149–150)

Actually in gonorrhea, there is no excrescence and no external growth. The main symptom of gonorrhea is purulent discharge through urethra. Excrescence or external growth at anogenital region occurs in (1) granuloma inguinale, (2) lymphogranuloma venereum, (3) condylomata, (4) condyloma acuminata.

Growth in anogenital region also occurs in other conditions like carcinoma but these are nonvenereal diseases. These diseases will not be discussed here because these are nonvenereal and Hahnemann described only venereal disease in relation to sycosis. There is a complete possibility that Hahnemann may have included nonvenereal diseases (like carcinoma, piles, etc. having external growth at anogenital region) in sycosis by erroneously presuming that these diseases are spread by coitus.

In summary, we can say Hahnemann included all venereal diseases into two groups, one where lesion is ulcerative or papular labeled as syphilitic miasm and second where lesion is like an external growth or discharge from urethra, labeled as sycosis miasm.

> Disease like granuloma inguinale begins as a papule which ulcerates and develops into a painless elevated zone may be mistaken for the primary chancre or condyloma latum of syphilis and when epithelial proliferation, resembling carcinoma in the genital or perianal region in a young subject should always raise the suspicion of granuloma inguinale. (Holmes, 1983b, p. 1000)

In granuloma inguinale, "Less common complications of the disease include deep ulceration, chronic cicatricial lesions, phimosis, lymphedema

Chapter forty two: Venereal diseases 167

and exuberant epithelial proliferation which grossly resemble carcinoma" (Holmes, 1983b, p. 1001).

This is my opinion that when diseases have such complications where external growth is a feature, Hahnemann must have included these in sycosis. In this discussion, there is no necessity to differentiate diseases into syphilis or sycosis. Our intention is to prove that diseases either part of syphilis or sycosis usually resolve spontaneously and gave the wrong message to Hahnemann and Kent, and other followers that they had been curing the disease by drugs having decillionth potency.

Granuloma inguinale which I have described already develops due to bacteria known as *Calymmatobacterium granulomatis.*

> Healing may occur at any stage or slow or rapid extension may continue intermittently and irregularly for years ... Temporary remissions may be followed by recrudescence which may occur in healed scars. When the lesions are extensive, cachexia may occur after a weary course of many years predisposing to death from intercurrent infection. (Roberts & Rook, 1979, p. 591)

> Diagnosis depends upon the finding of the Donovan bodies in scrapping or by the biopsy. It is important to exclude syphilis both by dark ground and by the serological examination. The lesions of granuloma inguinale in untreated cases after many months, tend to heal by themselves. When healing takes place, the scar may be atrophic and hypopigmented or hypertrophic. Some cases have been reported to develop malignancy. (Masani,1973, p. 304)

Next disease, lymphogranuloma venereum, is a sexually transmitted infection, caused by *Chlamydia trachomatis.* It is characterized by

> Infection of lymph channels and lymph nodes manifesting by bubo formation, ulcerations, enlargement of genital organs and rectal stricture. Fever, chills, headache and joint pains may also be present. Abscess formation with drainage of pus from the inguinal lymph nodes is usual. Later manifestations of disease include secondary ulceration and elephantiasis of genitals in both sexes, polypoid growths about the anus, and inflammation, ulceration and stricture of rectum. (Fleming, 1973, p. 242)

The most reliable method of diagnosis is isolation of chlamydia from aspirated bubo pus and by immuno-diagnostic tests. "Spontaneous healing usually occurs after several months leaving inguinal scars or granulomatous masses of varying size which persist for life" (Holmes, 1983c, p. 1085). "The untreated disease usually runs an average course of 6 to 8 weeks and may then resolve completely. Many cases are left with the sequelae of lymphatic obstruction and some show periodic recrudescences of activity for many years" (Nagington & Rook, 1979, p. 666). Clinically it is difficult to distinguish this disease from granuloma inguinal and genital tuberculosis.

> Chancroid (soft chancre) is an acute, specific, localized, self limiting, autoinoculable infectious disease. Disease is almost always acquired through sexual contact, initiated by an infection agent known as the Ducrey bacillus (a bacterium). It is characterized by painful ulceration at the site of inoculation usually on genitals and may be accompanied by purulent lymphadenitis. (Fleming, 1973, pp. 240–241)

"Disease of chancroid is self limited and systemic spread does not occur. Without treatment, genital ulcers and inguinal abscess have occasionally been reported to persist for years. Local pain is the most frequent complaint" (Eichmann, 1993, p. 2752).

"Condyloma acuminata or genital warts are usually asymptomatic. Small lesions appear as 1 to 2 mm white macules or papules. In most cases genital warts are numerous and appear in clusters. However solitary lesions may occur. Grape like or cauliflower like clustering does occur specially perianally" (Johnson, 1993, p. 1444). This disease for diagnosis has to be differentiated from condyloma lata, carcinomas, lichen planus, moles, seborrheic keratoses, cyst. It is a virus infection known as human papillomavirus. More than 60 types of HPV have been detected. "This virus infects the most epithelium of the anogenital region and results in a spectrum of lesions ranging from condyloma acuminata, intraepithelial neoplasia, and invasive squamous cell carcinoma" (Johnson, 1993, p. 1444).

Study of warts is important because sycosis miasm includes mainly warts and clinically similar diseases.

> Warts are benign neoplasms of the skin ... Warts are found in approximately 7 to 20 percent of the population, with the highest frequency in the early teenage years ... Person to person transmission by direct contact with wart tissue and indirectly by

Chapter forty two: Venereal diseases

> virus contamination through contaminated secre-
> tions or instruments may occur. Autoinoculation
> of viruses to contiguous or distant sites is
> frequent ... Warts are skin coloured, can be single
> or occur in multiple clusters and are often widely
> dispersed over the body. While warts may persist
> and spread within the same person for several years
> or may recur in an individual several years after a
> total remission. Most studies indicate that one third
> of warts are gone by 6 months and two thirds of
> warts will resolve spontaneously within a 2 year
> period ... During pregnancy warts may increase in
> size ... The development of anti wart antibodies has
> been correlated with clinical regression in patients
> or those with combined immunodeficiency warts
> may reappear ... Radical therapy of warts should
> be eschewed because most warts will eventually
> spontaneously disappear without leaving any scar.
> (Corey, 1983, pp. 1174–1175).

"Children with common warts may not require therapy. Studies of spontaneous regression of warts in children suggest that 2/3 will remit within 2 year with remaining verrucae continuing to resolve at this rate. However, new warts may appear while others are regressing" (Lowy & Androphy, 1993, p. 2619). "Neither the patient's age nor the number of warts present influences the course" (Nagington & Rook, 1979, p. 621). "Duration of genital warts varies from a few weeks to many years" (Nagington & Rook, 1979, p. 624).

When treatment part of the wart is considered, "Routine treatment of every wart is unnecessary and undesirable. The degree of disability must be carefully weighed against the discomfort or hazards of the proposed treatment and natural history of the wart and its probable spontaneous cure must be constantly borne in mind" (Nagington & Rook, 1979, p. 624).

> Most of the innumerable folk remedies for warts
> depend for their success on the tendency of warts to
> spontaneous resolution and possibly the influence
> of suggestion. It is widely believed that suggestion
> can cure warts. Both the probability of spontaneous
> cure and the possibility of influence by suggestion
> must be taken into account in planning and evaluat-
> ing any form of treatment. (Nagington & Rook, 1979,
> p. 624)

170   *Homeopathy*

It has been mentioned correctly, "As warts often disappear spontaneously, any treatment which is in use at the time will gain an undeserved reputation as a wart cure" (Rains & Ritchie, 1977, p. 101). It is also found that when one wart is treated by topical application, other warts present over the body disappear suddenly. In this phenomenon, immunity plays an important role.

Genital Herpes is a virus infection and is generally transmitted by sexual contact. Genital herpes is marked by clusters of small painful blisters on the genitals. After a few days, these blisters burst leaving small ulcers in their place. Almost all cases are marked by painful burning at the site of blister formation. Other relatively common symptoms include pain or burning during urination, discharge from the urethra or vagina, but these all tend to disappear within one or two weeks. If generalized symptoms appear, they diminish gradually over the first week of the infection. After the blisters burst, lesions usually heal in one to two weeks. Skin lesions last an average of 16–20 days, although the blisters disappear and the ulcers heal spontaneously. Many people have recurrent episodes of genital herpes varying in frequency from once a month to once every few years. People who suffer from herpes find that repeat herpes attacks tend to resolve completely after a few years (Masters et al., 1986, pp. 536–543).

Gonorrhea is a bacterial infection caused by *Neisseria gonorrhoeae*, a Gram-negative coccus. Gonorrhea in a male is characterized by purulent urethral discharge, dysuria, and frequent urination. Other local complications are inguinal lymphadenitis, edema of penis, and abscess. In homosexual men, anorectal and pharyngeal infections are common. In female dysuria, frequent urination, increased vaginal discharge, anorectal discomfort, midline low abdominal pain, and tenderness are common symptoms in gonorrhea. "Before antibiotic treatment became available, symptoms of urethritis persisted for an average of 8 weeks and unilateral epididymitis occurred in 5 to 10% untreated men" (Holmes, 1983a, p. 940). In homosexual men symptomatology of gonorrhea, "may subside without treatment, leaving a chronic asymptomatic carrier state" (Holmes, 1983a, p. 940). "Symptoms gradually resolve without treatment but it is not known how long patients remain infectious, the longer patients remain without treatment the more likely they are to develop complications" (Griffin et al., 1999, p. 187). "Acute symptoms of gonococcal urethritis in the female may subside spontaneously" (Holmes, 1983a, p. 941).

> From 1 to 3 percent of adults with gonococcal infection develop gonococcemia. The onset of gonococcemia is characterized by fever, polyarthralgias and papular, petechial, pustular, haemorrhagic or necrotic skin lesions. Wrists, fingers, knees and

Chapter forty two: Venereal diseases 171

ankles most often involve joints. Without treatment, the duration of gonococcemia is variable, the systemic manifestations of bacteremia may subside spontaneously within a week. (Holmes, 1983a, p. 941)

External hemorrhoids are not sexually transmitting diseases. Some homeopaths include this disease in sycosis.

A thrombosed external hemorrhoid appears suddenly and is very painful. The haematoma is usually situated in a lateral region of the anal margin. In the majority of cases resolution or fibrosis occurs. Indeed this condition has been called a five day painful, self curing lesion. (Rains & Ritchie, 1977, p. 1067)

Condyloma lata are skin lesions of secondary syphilis. These lesions also subside spontaneously.

At the time of Hahnemann, differential diagnosis of various sexually transmitted diseases was not possible. "Until the nineteenth century, genital warts were believed to be a form of syphilis and gonorrhea" (Lowy & Androphy, 1993, p. 2611). This mistake was made by Hahnemann and Kent. All diseases that were presumed due to syphilis and sycosis miasm usually resolved spontaneously. This gave false observation to Hahnemann and Kent that they had been curing these diseases.

As written by Hahneman,

The gonorrhea dependent on the fig wart miasm as well as the above mentioned excrescence (the whole sycosis) are cured most surely and most thoroughly through the internal use of thuja which in this case is homeopathic in a dose of a few pellets as large as poppy seeds, moistened with the dilution potentized to the decillionth degree and when these have exhausted their action after fifteen, twenty, thirty, forty days alternating with just as small a dose of nitric acid diluted to the decillionth degree which must be allowed to act as long a time in order to remove the gonorrhea and the excrescence – the whole sycosis. (Hahnemann, 1999, p. 151)

In this way, Hahnemann made the wrong concept of homeopathy.

References

Corey, L. (1983). Warts & molluscum contagiosum. In R. G. Petersdorf, R. D. Adams, E. Braunwald, K. J. Isselbacher, J. B. Martin, & J. D. Wilson (Eds.), *Harrison's principle of internal medicine* (10th ed., pp. 1174–1180). New Delhi, India: McGraw hill.

Eichmann, A. R. (1993). Chancroid. In T. B. Fitzpatrick, A. Z. Risen, K. Wolff, I. M. Greenberg, & K. F. Austin (Eds.), *Dermatology in general medicine* (4th ed., Vol 2, pp. 2749–2752). New York, NY, NY: McGraw-Hill.

Fleming, W. L. (1973). Venereal diseases. In P. E. Sartwell, & E. Sartwell (Eds.), *Maxcy-Rosenau-preventive medicine and public health* (10th ed., pp. 229–246). New York, NY: Appleton-Century-Crofts (A publishing division of Prentice Hall).

Griffin, G. E., Sissons, J. G. P., Chiodini, P. L., Mitchell, D. M. (1999). Diseases due to infection. In C. Haslett, E. R. Chillers, J. A. A. Hunter, & N. A. Boon (Eds.), *Davidson's principles and practice of medicine* (18th ed., pp. 56–190). Edinburgh, United Kingdom: Churchill Livingstone.

Hahnemann, S. (1999). *The chronic diseases (theoretical part)* (Reprint ed.). New Delhi, India: B Jain Publishers.

Holmes, K. K. (1983a). Gonococcal infection. In R. G. Petersdorf, R. D. Adams, E. Braunwald, K. J. Isselbacher, J. B. Martin, & J. D. Wilson (Eds.), *Harrison's principle of internal medicine* (10th ed., pp. 939–945). New Delhi, India: McGraw Hill.

Holmes, K. K. (1983b). Granuloma inguinale. In R. G. Petersdorf, R. D. Adams, E. Braunwald, K. J. Isselbacher, J. B. Martin, & J. D. Wilson (Eds.), *Harrison's principle of internal medicine* (10th ed., pp. 1000–1001). New Delhi, India: McGraw Hill.

Holmes, K. K. (1983c). Lymphogranuloma venereum. In J. D. Wilson (Ed.), *Harrison's principle of internal medicine* (10th ed., pp. 1084–1086). New Delhi, India: McGraw Hill.

Johnson, R. A. (1993). Diseases & disorders of anogenitalia of males. In T. B. Fitzpatrick, A. Z. Risen, K. Wolff, I. M. Greenberg, & K. F. Austins (Eds.), *Dermatology in general medicine* (4th ed., Vol. 1, pp. 1417–1462). New York, NY: McGraw-Hill.

Lowy, D. R., & Androphy, E. R. (1993). Warts. In T. B. Fitzpatrick, A. Z. Risen, K. Wolff, I. M. Greenberg, & K. F. Austin (Eds.), *Dermatology in general medicine* (4th ed, Vol. 2, pp. 2611–2620). New York, NY: McGraw-Hill.

Masani, K. M. (1973). *A textbook of gynaecology* (7th ed.). Bombay, India: Popular Prakashan.

Masters, W. H., Johnson, V. E., & Kolodny, R. C. (1986). *Masters & Johnson on sex and human loving.* Mumbai, India: Jaico Publishing House.

Nagington, J., & Rook, A. (1979). Virus and related infection. In A. Rook, D. S. Wilkinson, & F. J. G. Ebling (Eds.), *Textbook of dermatology* (3rd ed., Vol. 1, pp. 607–676). Oxford, United Kingdom: Blackwell Scientific Publication.

Rains, A. J. H., & Ritchie, H. D. (1977). *Bailey & love's short practice of surgery* (17th ed.). London, United Kingdom: H. K. Levi's & Co Ltd.

Roberts, S. O. B., & Rook, A. (1979). Bacterial infection. In A. Rook, D. S. Wilkinson, & F. J. G. Ebling (Eds.). *Textbook of dermatology* (3rd ed., Vol. 1, pp. 541–606). Oxford, United Kingdom: Blackwell Scientific Publication.

chapter forty three

Chancroid and chancre

Basic concept of homeopathy – forty three

It had been thought previously that syphilis always follows on the destruction of chancre by local applications and allopathic drugs modify acute diseases into chronic diseases that become very troublesome to people.

Argument

Development of knowledge is a continuous process. Even in medical science, what was acceptable in 1900 has been discarded today. "In 1892 Guanieri gave the first clear description of small-pox, what he believed to be a parasitic protozoan" (Ruhrah, 1913, p. 41). But today we know with absolute proof that it was a virus infection. Previously, local treatment of the chancre was indicated in allopathy (Gottheil, 1913, p. 422), which was opposed by Hahnemann but in modern medical science at present no local treatment is indicated in syphilis and gonorrhea.

When medical concepts of 1900 are not acceptable today on the basis of new inventions and discoveries, then how old unscientific and hypothetical concepts of homeopathy can be accepted today? I am giving some more examples of how Hahnemann made wrong conclusions. Hahnemann quoted John hunter and Fabre. John Hunter says, "Not one patient out of fifteen will escape syphilis if the chancre is destroyed by mere external applications" (Hahnemann, 1999, p. 155). Fabre declares, "Syphilis always follows on the destruction of the chancre by local applications" (Hahnemann, 1999, p. 155). These were the wrong conclusions. Today we know even without localized destruction of chancre, syphilis will remain and spread in the body. Appearance of the secondary stage of syphilis is not related in any way to the local destruction of chancre.

Hahnemann writes at one place, "I have never, in my practice of more than fifty years seen any trace of the venereal disease break out so long as the chancre remained untouched in its place even if this were a space of several years" (Hahnemann, 1999, p. 156).

It was actually chancroid not chancre, which has been wrongly understood as chancre by Hahnemann. Because "During medieval time chancroid was not distinguished from the initial lesion of syphilis but it was not until 1850 that soft chancre was distinguished from the initial lesion

DOI: 10.1201/9781003228622-43

173

174   *Homeopathy*

of syphilis and later designated chancroid (chancre like)" (Fleming, 1973, p. 241). In some cases of chancroid, "Untreated chancroid ulcers persist for long periods of time and often progress" (Austen, 1983, p. 374).

Hahnemann also said at various places that allopathic drugs modify acute diseases into chronic diseases (Hahnemann, 1921/1996, p. 98) and chronic diseases that are produced by allopathy are very troublesome to people (Hahnemann, 1921/1996, p. 100). "Chronic medical dyscrasia so often produced by allopathic bungling along with the natural disease left uncured by it require a much longer time for their recovery often indeed, are they incurable" (Hahnemann, 1921/1993, p. 216). Hahnemann also mentioned that allopathic drugs when removed external manifestations or discharge, disease redirected internally from the surface and creates various systemic symptoms. Hahnemann repeatedly mentioned that allopathic drugs are very dangerous. Hahnemann was right because, during his time, antibiotics had not been discovered. Metals and their compounds were used in various diseases and these compounds were very toxic; that's why they are not used today.

In spontaneously curable diseases, allopathic drugs developed various toxic manifestations, while homeopathic drugs were totally harmless. Homeopathic drugs have no effect as well as no side effects. Spontaneous curable diseases will be cured without the help of any drug. With the help of homeopathic drugs, Hahnemann protected the population from toxic manifestations of old allopathic procedures.

References

Austen, K. F. (1983). Diseases of immediate type of hypersensitivity. In R. G. Petersdorf, R. D. Adams, E. Braunwald, K. J. Isselbacher, J. B. Martin, & J. D. Wilson (Eds.), *Harrison's principle of internal medicine* (10th ed., pp. 372–377). New Delhi, India: McGraw Hill.

Fleming, W. L. (1973). Venereal diseases. In P. E. Sartwell, & E. Sartwell (Eds.), *Maxcy-Rosenau-preventive medicine and public health* (10th ed., pp. 229–246). New York, NY: Appleton-Century-Crofts (A publishing division of Prentice Hall).

Gottheil, E. S. (1913). The general & special treatment of syphilis. In F. Forchheimer (Ed.), *Therapeutics of internal diseases* (Vol 2, pp. 361–437). Sydney, Australia: Butterworth & Co.

Hahnemann, S. (1993). *Organon of medicine* (6th ed.) (W.Boericke, Trans.). New Delhi, India: B. Jain Publishers. (Original work published in 1921).

Hahnemann, S. (1996). *Organon of medicine* (6th ed.) (P. Devi, Trans.). New Delhi, India: B. Jain Publishers. (Original work published in 1921).

Hahnemann, S. (1999). *The chronic diseases (theoretical part)* (Reprint ed.). New Delhi, India: B Jain Publishers.

Ruhrah, J. (1913). Smallpox. In F. Forchheimer (Ed.), *Therapeutics of internal diseases* (Vol 2, pp. 40–53). Sydney, Australia: Butterworth & Co.

chapter forty four

Allopathic drugs suppress symptoms

Basic concept of homeopathy – forty four

Allopathic drugs suppress symptoms, redirect them internally, and create various systemic disturbances. By suppression of psora, syphilis, and sycosis after the administration of allopathic injections, many types of disease symptoms are produced.

Argument

Hahnemann had one more typical argument about the suppression of external symptoms. Hahnemann was of the opinion that all external symptoms and externally localized lesions are part of internal diseases. Hahnemann said that when external symptoms or externally localized lesions are removed by internally used homeopathic drugs, then it is alright. But when externally localized lesions or symptoms are removed by internally used allopathic drugs, it is wrong. He also said, "When allopathic drugs are used, they suppress symptoms, then disease redirects internally and creates various disorders".

Hahnemann thought that homeopathic drugs cure symptoms, while allopathic drugs suppress symptoms and create systemic disturbances. How did Hahnemann reach such a conclusion? Homeopathic drugs actually do not cure the disease and never produce side effects, while allopathic drugs used in the sexually transmitted disease, at the time of Hahnemann, were very toxic irrespective of therapeutic effect. "Many chemicals are toxic to cell ... Effect upon cells may be nonselective and cells of the host as well as invading bacteria may be killed" (Krantz & Carr, 1965, pp. 205–206).

"Mercuric metallic ions get adsorbed on the surface of bacterium and then enter and coagulate the protoplasm ... Mercury-like arsenic combines with sulfhydryl groups in the bacterial cell thus interfering with cellular metabolism" (Iswariah & Guruswami, 1972, p. 626). "Mercury, while not being an active spirochaeticide, accumulates in the syphilitic lesions and inhibits the development of organisms. But coincidental with such a spirochaetostatic effect appear symptoms of chronic mercurialism.

DOI: 10.1201/9781003228622-44

176 *Homeopathy*

Bismuth took the place of mercury until the development of penicillin treatment" (Iswariah & Guruswami, 1972, p. 819). In the pre-antibiotic era, "Antimony compounds were the standby in the treatment of the disease-granuloma venereum" (Iswariah & Guruswami, 1972, p. 740).

> Results with mercury treatment in syphilis were far from satisfactory for the attendant mercurialism coupled with doubtful result within a few decades of its birth, arsenic treatment has become obsolete in syphilis. Toxic complications during the necessary prolonged arsenic therapy often claimed as high a mortality as the disease itself. Bismuth, introduced in 1922 as a substitute for mercury as a complement to arsenic ... Penicillin today has been proved to be curative in syphilis beyond any claim of the earlier drugs. (Iswariah & Guruswami, 1972, p. 626)

> Bismuth immobilized the spirochetes (Causative organism of syphilis) rendering them noninfectious. Bismuth may, therefore, be stated to prevent the spread and multiplication of spirochetes and depresses the disease to a point where the degree of resistance already existing in the body can control the infection. (Iswariah & Guruswami, 1972, p. 748)

"Unlike the organic arsenicals which have fallen out in complete disuse in the therapy of syphilis, bismuth and its compounds are still in use as an adjunct to penicillin therapy in latent syphilis and cardiovascular syphilis" (Iswariah & Guruswami, 1972, p. 749). "Antimony and potassium tartrate was first used in the treatment of granuloma inguinale. The injections are given at intervals of 2 to 3 days, 10 to 12 injections may clear the lesions sufficiently" (Beckman, 1943, p. 719).

In allopathy, chemicals were used in the treatment of various sexually transmitted diseases at the time of Hahnemann. We also know that differential diagnosis was also not clear at that time. Syphilis may have been diagnosed as gonorrhea and chancroid may have been diagnosed as chancre. Now we also know that these chemicals were used in sexually transmitted diseases in high concentrations repeatedly in the form of injections and are highly toxic. Toxic complications during the necessary prolonged arsenic therapy are often claimed as high a mortality as the disease itself. Spirochaeticidal concentration of mercury produces symptoms of chronic mercurialism. Hahnemann said that allopathic drugs suppressed the disease, which produced various internal ailments.

Chapter forty four: Allopathic drugs suppress symptoms 177

Homeopaths say that by suppression of psora, syphilis, and sycosis after the administration of allopathic injections, many types of disease symptoms are produced. Gradually the liver, spleen, and other abdominal organs are damaged. Abdominal problems are seen. Tubercular and other chronic problems are also developed due to this suppression (Ghatak, 1938, pp. 80–82).

From the above discussion, it is clear that administration of allopathic drugs does not produce new disease symptoms by suppressing external manifestations. Allopathic drugs cured some sexually transmitted diseases at the time of Hahnemann but produced many toxic symptoms. These toxic symptoms were misunderstood by Hahnemann as systemic pathology created by the suppression of external symptoms and redirected them internally.

References

Beckman, H. (1943). *Treatment in general practice* (4th ed.). Philadelphia, PA: W. B. Saunders Company.

Ghatak, N. (1938). *Cause and cure of chronic diseases* (4th ed.) (C. S. Pathak, Trans.).Kolkata,India: Dr. S.M. Bhattacharya. (Original work published in 1931).

Iswariah, V., & Guruswami, M. N. (1972). *David-Iswariah-Guruswami's pharmacology and pharmacotherapy* (7th ed.). Madras, India: P. Varadachary and Co.

Krantz, J. C., & Carr, C. J. (1965). *The pharmacological principles of medical practice* (6th ed.). Baltimore, MD: Williams and Wilkins Company.

chapter forty five

Fig-wart diseases and gonorrhea

Basic concept of homeopathy – forty five

Fig-wart disease is the result of suppression of gonorrhea by allopathic treatment. Suppression of symptoms increases severity of disease. Kent concluded that allopathic drugs suppressed gonorrhea in male and after marriage this suppressed gonorrhea transmitted to females and caused many symptoms.

Argument

Kent said,

> There are two kinds of gonorrhea, one that is essentially chronic, having no disposition to recovery … one that is acute, and has a tendency to recover after a few weeks or months … The acute may really and truly be called a gonorrhea because about all there is of it is this discharge … The suppression of acute gonorrhea cannot bring on the constitutional symptoms called sycosis. It can not be followed by fig-warts, nor constitutional states such as anemia. But while constitutional symptoms cannot follow the suppression of acute miasm, they will follow suppression of the chronic miasm and become very serious. Most of the cases of true sycosis that are brought before the physician at the present time are those that have been suppressed. (Kent, 1993, p. 144)

Kent said that fig-wart disease is the result of suppression of gonorrhea by allopathic treatment. It is absolutely wrong. Fig-wart disease is a viral infection and gonorrhea is a bacterial infection, both diseases are different. It is not possible that suppression of gonorrhea results in fig-wart disease. This is an entirely different matter that both diseases can exist together. Surprisingly, it has been found by observations that other venereal disease and fig-wart disease usually coexist together.

DOI: 10.1201/9781003228622-45

179

"In the past, genital warts were termed gonorrheal or venereal warts. These terms are misleading and should not be used, although such patients quite often have associated venereal disease" (King et al., 1980, p. 363). This coexistence of both diseases confused Hahnemann and Kent who gave false statements that suppression of gonorrhea (venereal disease) produces fig-wart disease. Kent and Hahnemann repeatedly said that suppression of symptoms increases severity of disease and after that internal organs are affected. It is not correct.

Collection of pus, rotten tissue, abnormal growth, stone in important organs have to be removed from the body and such removal is not a part of only symptomatic improvement, it is an actual cure. Removal of pain and fever only are parts of symptomatic improvement. We should not confuse these two concepts.

Kent said, "In a year or eighteen months after marriage with uterine trouble, with ovarian disease, with abdominal troubles, with all sorts of complaints peculiar to the woman and it has been found that her husband had two three attack of gonorrhea that were treated with allopathic drugs" (Kent, 1993, p. 146). Kent concluded that allopathic drugs suppressed gonorrhea in male and after marriage this suppressed gonorrhea transmitted to females and caused many mentioned symptoms. Kent also said, "Suppression of gonorrhea leads to anaemia" (Kent, 1993, p. 146).

Kent described many symptoms due to suppression of gonorrhea. Kent said,

> Sometimes it is so very severe in form and the trouble comes so soon after the suppression that there can be no doubt even in the mind of the man himself, that the trouble he is now suffering from relates to the suppression of that discharge. Sometimes they are latent and develop very gradually and the blood becomes affected and gradually increasing anaemia comes and the patient being pallid and waxy. (Kent, 1993, p. 146)

Kent said that diseases of the uterus and ovary, abdominal troubles, and all sorts of complaints peculiar to the woman are due to suppressed gonorrhea. It was only the imagination and hypothesis of Kent. There are hundreds of causes of these symptoms. Without isolation of bacteria, serological tests, and other investigations, nothing can be said. Kent mentioned suppression of gonorrhea in male and after 1 year from suppression, his wife suffered from many symptoms which Kent said were due to gonorrhea, transmitted from husband. Here I say that symptomatology in females was definitely due to something other than gonorrhea because at

Chapter forty five: Fig-wart diseases and gonorrhea   *181*

that time accurate diagnostic facilities were not available and there was no knowledge about other diseases of females. We also know today that "in most cases of gonorrhea there are few systemic symptoms beyond malaise and a slight headache" (Beckman, 1953, p. 708). How can all gynecological problems of females be correlated with gonorrhea? Such correlation is unscientific and baseless. In gonorrhea we also know, "Acute symptoms of gonococcal urethritis in the female may subside spontaneously" (Holmes, 1983, p. 941). "Symptoms gradually resolve without treatment but it is not known how long patients remain infectious" (Griffin et al., 1999, p. 187). That's why without confirming diagnosis of disease such type of hypothesis should not be accepted. At the time of Hahnemann and Kent, there were confusions in diagnosis of disease. This confusion and wrong diagnosis created misnomer and wrong hypotheses which are being accepted by homeopaths and their followers, e.g., "Until the nineteenth century genital warts were believed to be a form of syphilis or gonorrhea" (Lowy & Androphy, 1993, p. 2611). Such wrong concepts are mainly responsible for the origin of homeopathy.

According to Kent, sycosis means suppressed gonorrhea and fig-wart disease is a sycotic trouble. Kent writes,

> A man who has gone from ten to fifteen years with this sycotic trouble. He is waxy, subject to various kinds of fig-warts, his lips are pale and his ears almost transparent, ... he has various kinds of manifestations ... that we call symptoms ... The trouble may have manifested itself in other mucous membranes of the body and thus saved the man from his waxiness. He is not so pallid when the condition becomes busy in another region. These catarrhal manifestations may be catarrhal conditions of the eyes but are commonly catarrhs of the nose. It is not an uncommon thing for a nasal catarrh to be sycotic and to have existed only since the gonorrhea was suppressed. The catarrh is located in the nose and posterior nares with thick copious discharge. (Kent, 1993, pp. 146–147)

Kent further explained that suppression of gonorrheal discharge creates internal pathology and gives rise to many symptoms. When treatment has been done by homeopathic drug, suppressed gonorrhea discharge should be brought externally from the nose. "When the constitution is vigorous enough it will keep up the discharge in spite of the different specific remedies that have been administered but in constitutions that are feeble

182   *Homeopathy*

diseases are easily driven to the centre, leaving the outermost parts of man" (Kent, 1993, p. 147). In this way what homeopathy says, discharge should come back externally. Kent writes, "So it is often the case that a man with a thick yellowish-green discharge from the nose after a dose of calcarea which is an antisycotic, one of the deepest in character, has his old discharge, brought back" (Kent, 1993, p. 147). Kent also said, "If the catarrh does not come on soon the constitution is too weak for the catarrh to represent the disease and it will be represented on deeper tissues. Bright's disease may come, breaking down of the lungs, breaking down of the liver, rheumatic affection of the worst form finally killing the patient" (Kent, 1993, p. 148).

Kent said that if gonorrhea discharge is not coming outside the body in catarrhal form, it will damage many internal organs in male and female. Kent writes,

> Sometimes in the man it does not take the catarrhal form but produces inflammation of the testes or it may affect the rectum. Again if you go to the bedside of a man who has used strong injections for the purpose of suppressing a gonorrheal discharge and you find him in bed writhing and turning, tossing, twisting with the pain and the only relief for him is to keep in continual motion, the pains are tremendous, they are rending and tearing from head to foot. (Kent, 1993, p. 148)

Kent and Hahnemann both said that suppression of gonorrheal discharge is responsible for creating many new signs and symptoms of internal pathology. And I say, it was the wrong observation of Hahnemann and Kent. The signs and symptoms of internal pathology were due to toxicity of allopathic drugs given for the treatment of sexually transmitted disease.

I have written previously that at the time of Hahnemann compounds of mercury, arsenic and bismuth were used as chemotherapeutic agents. The standard method of treatment was "To administer a variable number of neoarsphenamine and to supplement these with intramuscular injections of mercury or bismuth. The whole treatment extends over a period of two years" (Clark, 1938, p. 614). "Regular administration of arsenic in any soluble form does not produce tolerance but on the contrary produces cumulative poisoning. The arsenic retained is distributed throughout the body" (Clark, 1938, p. 618).

Mercury was the first drug to be used as a specific disinfectant.

> Satisfactory results are only produced by mercury after prolonged action and the minimum efficient

Chapter forty five: Fig-wart diseases and gonorrhea 183

> therapeutic concentration of mercury closely approaches the toxic concentration ... Mercury is excreted very slowly and hence has a marked cumulative action ... This metal was stored in various organs and particularly in the kidney and liver ... After a course of mercurial treatment the body gets rid of the mercury very slowly and small quantities continue to be excreted for three months after the last dose has been given. (Clark, 1938, pp. 626–628)

Hahnemann writes, "Mercury has been used internally" (Hahnemann, 1999, pp. 15–19). Administration of these metallic compounds may have cured the diseases or diseases were cured spontaneously but this is certain that these drugs must have produced many symptoms due to toxicity which Hahnemann and Kent said, originated due to suppression of gonorrhea. Some toxicity of these metallic compounds appeared on the surface like increased discharge through mouth and nose that has been called by Hahnemann and Kent as reappearance of discharge through mouth and nose. "Salivation and gingivitis are the first symptoms of mercurial poisoning. The salivation is often very marked and several litres of saliva may be secreted a day" (Clark, 1938, p. 632). "The mucous membranes of the throat, nose become Inflamed with an associated conjunctivitis in chronic arsenic poisoning" (Krantz & Carr, 1965, p. 164). "Iodine and its salts are the second remedy for syphilis. Abundant nasal discharge, swelling of the nasal and ocular mucosa, fever, headache and general malaise may form a true iodic influenza" (Gottheil, 1913, p. 406). Kent emphasized that nasal catarrh and catarrh of other mucous membranes are due to suppression of gonorrhea but now we can say, it is due to toxicity of drugs used by allopathic doctors.

Arsenic that was used by allopathic doctors also causes, "perspiration, excessive salivation, sweating, stomatitis, sore throat, coryza, lacrimation" (Klaassen, 1980, p. 1631), and such type of action of allopathic drugs confused Hahnemann and Kent who said these are symptoms of suppressed gonorrhea which is coming externally by homeopathic drugs. At the time of Hahnemann, there was no knowledge about toxicity of these metallic compounds and there were no pharmacokinetic and pharmacodynamic studies of these compounds. As mentioned rightly,

> There have been epidemics of mercury poisoning among wildlife and human populations in many countries ... With very few exceptions and for numerous reasons such outbreaks were

184 *Homeopathy*

> misdiagnosed for months or even years … Factors
> in these tragic delays included the insidious onset
> of the affliction, vagueness of early clinical signs
> and the medical profession's unfamiliarity with the
> disease. (Gerstner & Huff, 1977, pp. 491–526)

Kent writes, "It is often the case that a man with a thick yellowish green discharge from the nose after a dose of calcarea, which is an antisycotic, one of the deepest in character has his old discharge brought back" (Kent, 1993, p. 147). We know from the knowledge of chemistry that many compounds of mercury and arsenic are colored. "In arsenic poisoning there is high coloured, bloody stool" (Modi, 1975, p. 526). "In chronic arsenic poisoning gums become red and soft and the tongue is coated with a thin white silvery fur" (Modi, 1975, p. 529). "Gingivitis due to mercury poisoning may be due to mercury lining precipitated in the gums as mercury sulphide by the sulfurated hydrogen present in the mouth" (Clark, 1938, p. 632). "Mercuric sulphide is obtained as a black precipitate, turns red on sublimation and gradually also turns red and crystalline" (Soni, 1981, p. 2.221). Kent observed colored nasal discharge after homeopathic drug administration and said old discharge is being brought back. It was wrong. Actually, it was toxicity of metallic compounds, administered by allopathic doctors.

Kent described manifestations of suppressed gonorrhea,

> Patient being pallid and waxy, anemia comes,
> patient has various kinds of manifestation, catarrh
> conditions of the eyes and nose, breaking down of
> the lungs, breaking down of the liver, Bright's disease may come, rheumatic affection of the worst
> form finally killing the patient and he becomes
> anemic, tremendous pain, tendons will begin to
> contract and they will shorten the muscles of the
> calves, the muscles of the thighs will become so sore
> that they cannot be touched or handled, sometimes
> there is infiltration of the muscles and hardness and
> this soreness extends to the bottom of the feet so
> that it is impossible for the patient to walk. (Kent,
> 1993, pp. 144–151)

These manifestations that were described by Kent due to suppression of gonorrhea were in fact manifestations of chronic toxicity of metallic compounds used for allopathic treatment. Abdominal pain, dry and congested throat symptoms of neuritis are more pronounced, severe cramps

Chapter forty five: Fig-wart diseases and gonorrhea   185

in the muscles which are extremely tender on pressure, patient is very restless and cannot sleep and there may be death. In cases which end in recovery, chronic peripheral neuritis may persist. These are subacute toxicities of arsenic. Chronic toxicity of arsenic has the following features, malaise, salivation, colicky pain, constipation, vomiting of glairy mucus tinged with bile; gums are reds soft, cough with expectoration; liver and kidney are damaged; epithelioma may develop in 20% of these cases; tingling and numbness of the extremities, hyperesthesia of the skin, marked tenderness and cramps of the muscles arthralgia and circumscribed edema, aplastic anemia, peripheral neuritis, muscular atrophy, etc. (Modi, 1975, p. 530).

Compounds of mercury when taken internally for a prolonged period symptoms begin to appear.

> These are nausea, digestive disturbances, colicky pain, vomiting, diarrhoea. Salivation is a constant symptom which is accompanied by foul breath, swollen and painful salivary glands, inflamed and ulcerated gums, which occasionally present a brownish blue line at their junction with teeth ... rarely necrosis of the jaw develops ... brownish deposit of mercury through the cornea on the anterior lens capsule ... cough with bloody expectoration, suffers from general wasting, anaemia, and chronic nephritis, and dies from exhaustion. (Modi, 1975, pp. 549–550)

> Sazerac & Lavaditi (1922) showed that bismuth was a powerful spirochaeticide, the drug rapidly attained popularity as a substitute for mercury in the treatment of syphilis ... Bismuth salts when used in the treatment of syphilis are always given intramuscularly ... The toxic actions produced by bismuth are very similar to those produced by mercury. Blue gum line and salivation also occurs. More serious effects are malaise, and loss of weight, diarrhoea albuminuria, dermatitis and jaundice. (Clark, 1938, p. 632)

Now we know symptoms of suppressed gonorrhea are the same as toxic symptoms produced by metallic compounds used in sexually transmitting diseases. There is nothing like suppression of disease by allopathic drugs. It is also wrong that homeopathic drugs bring back the manifestation of disease.

186 *Homeopathy*

Either diseases had been cured spontaneously or diseases were cured by metallic compounds. Administered metallic compounds produced toxic symptomatology for which Kent said symptoms are coming back by homeopathic drugs. Later on, toxic symptomatology was resolved gradually then Kent said, "This is the cure done by homeopathy".

Actually, homeopathic drugs have no effect, no side effects, and no therapeutic utility.

References

Beckman, H. (1953). *Pharmacology in clinical practice*. London, United Kingdom: W. B. Saunders and Company.

Clark, A. J. (1938). *Applied pharmacology* (6th ed.). London, United Kingdom: J. and A. Churchill LTD.

Gerstner, H. B., & Huff, J. E. (1977). Clinical toxicology of mercury. *Journal of Toxicology and Environment Health*, 2(3), 491–526. doi: 10.1080/1528739770952945.

Gottheil, E. S. (1913). The general and special treatment of syphilis. In F. Forchheimer (Ed.). *Therapeutics of internal diseases* (Vol. 2, pp. 361–437). Sydney, Australia: Butterworth and Co.

Griffin, G. E., Sissons, J. G. P., Chiodini, P. L., & Mitchell, D. M. (1999). Diseases due to infection. In C. Haslett, E. R. Chillers, J. A. A. Hunter, & N. A. Boon (Eds.), *Davidson's principles and practice of medicine* (18th ed., pp. 56–190). Edinburgh, United Kingdom: Churchill Livingstone.

Hahnemann, S. (1999). *The chronic diseases (theoretical part)* (Reprint ed.). New Delhi, India: B Jain Publishers.

Holmes, K. K. (1983). Gonococcal infection. In R. G. Petersdorf, R. D. Adams, E. Braunwald, K. J. Isselbacher, J. B. Martin, & J. D. Wilson (Eds.), *Harrison's principle of internal medicine* (10th ed., pp. 939–945). New Delhi, India: McGraw-Hill.

Kent, J. T. (1993). *Lectures on homeopathic philosophy*. Delhi, India: B. Jain Publishers.

King, A., Nicol, C., & Rodin, P. (1980). *Venereal diseases* (4th ed.). London, United Kingdom: ELBS and Bailliere Tindall.

Klaassen, C. D. (1980). Heavy metals and heavy metals antagonists. In A. G. Gilman, L. Goodman, & A. Gilman (Eds.), *Goodman and Gilman's pharmacological basis of therapeutics* (6th ed., pp. 1615–1637). New York, NY: Macmillan.

Krantz, J. C., & Carr, C. J. (1965). *The pharmacological principles of medical practice* (6th ed.). Baltimore, MD: Williams and Wilkins Company.

Lowy, D. R., & Androphy, E. R. (1993). Warts. In T. B. Fitzpatrick, A. Z. Risen, K. Wolff, I. M. Greenberg, & K. F. Austin (Eds.), *Dermatology in general medicine* (4th ed., Vol. 2, pp. 2611–2620). New York, NY: McGraw-Hill.

Modi, N. J. (1975). *Textbook of medical jurisprudence and toxicology* (9th ed.). Bombay, India: N.M. Tripathi, Publisher.

Soni, P. L. (1981). *Textbook of inorganic chemistry* (13th ed.). New Delhi, India: Sultan Chand and Sons Publications.

chapter forty six

Suppressed manifestations must come back

Basic concept of homeopathy – forty six

Suppressed manifestations must come back and they will come back under appropriate homeopathic treatment.

Argument

Statements of homeopathy on different subjects are interrelated. They cannot be isolated. They are interdependent also. That's why arguments against different basic concepts of homeopathy are also interrelated. No clear-cut demarcation is possible and chances of repetition are there. So for the argument against the basic concept of homeopathy forty six, please also study argument forty five.

Kent writes about syphilis that suppressed manifestations must come back and they will come back under appropriate homeopathic treatment. I have written previously that the periodicity of recurrence of syphilitic symptoms before spontaneous cure presented the false impression that suppressed manifestations are coming back. Another cause of this false opinion was toxicity of allopathic drugs used in the treatment of sexually transmitting diseases. It had been said that mercury and arsenic suppressed manifestations of syphilis which should come back for actual cure. For treatment of syphilis, arsenic and mercury were given.

> Arsenic has a marked toxic action on the heart, liver and kidneys. If the patient survives the gastrointestinal irritation, he may die later from injury to the vital organs. In chronic poisoning the first visible effect is a discolouration of the skin which may vary from grey to brown and keratosis occurs in the palms and soles. Conjunctivitis and laryngitis are common. Occasionally jaundice and cirrhosis are produced. (Clark, 1938, p. 620)

DOI: 10.1201/9781003228622-46

188   *Homeopathy*

> Jaundice may appear a few days after the administration of an organic arsenical but this type of early jaundice is rarely fatal. It is uncertain to what extent jaundice occurring during treatment is due to the drug or to the disease. Syphilis can cause considerable damage to the liver and jaundice may occur in untreated cases. Occasionally jaundice develops a considerable time after the treatment has been concluded. In this case also it is uncertain whether the condition is due to drug or to the disease. (Clark, 1938, p. 623)

Toxicity of mercuric compounds and syphilis give more or less similar clinical manifestations, that's why it is not easy to decide that it is drug toxicity or syphilitic manifestations.

Gottheil has written rightly in 1913,

> A too prolonged administration of the drug occasions a toxic chloro anemia shown by general lassitude, insomnia, loss of weight and even cachexia that may be readily confounded with the similar condition incident to early syphilitic poisoning or extensive late lesions, complicated with secondary infections. The differentiation between the two is not easy to make by watching the results of treatment. Every once in a while there comes into my wards at the city hospital a patient in a deplorable general condition emaciated, bedridden, covered with ulcerative gummata or with bone or internal syphilis ... Sometimes this patient is suffering from syphilis and septic infection and then mercury and other antisyphilitic remedies act like a charm. All the symptoms improve rapidly and the drug properly administered not only cures the symptoms of active diseases but is an absolute tonic and reconstituent. But sometimes the patient has had vigorous treatment before and gets progressively worse under mercury, iodine or arsenic. Stop all internal medication for such a patient, save mild local measures, put his bed where he can have plenty of light and air, give him as much milk and the most nutritious diet possible and behold improvement starts at once and progresses rapidly ... such patients with

Chapter forty six: Suppressed manifestations must come back 189

> the most extensive tertiary ulceration have everyone
> healed in a month under nothing but a simple boric
> acid w.e.f. dressing and gaining weight at the rate
> of a pound a day. They are suffering from chronic
> hydrargyrum rather than from syphilis. (Gottheil,
> 1913, pp. 383–384)

With this statement of Frederick, it is very clear that manifestations of syphilis were removed but toxic manifestations of metallic compounds appeared. In these patients, nothing should be given. Patients would be alright when toxic manifestations subside. These toxic manifestations were also labeled as suppressed manifestations releasing due to homeopathic treatment as said by Kent, "Bringing out external manifestations upon his body somewhere" (Kent, 1993, p. 143).

References

Clark, A. J. (1938). *Applied pharmacology* (6th ed.). London, United Kingdom: J. & A. Churchill LTD.

Gottheil, E. S. (1913). The general and special treatment of syphilis. In F. Forchheimer (Ed.), *Therapeutics of internal diseases* (Vol. 2, pp. 361–437). Sydney, Australia: Butterworth and Co.

Kent, J. T. (1993). *Lectures on homeopathic philosophy*. Delhi, India: B. Jain Publishers.

chapter forty seven

Psora and spiritualism

Basic concept of homeopathy – forty seven

Psora is the most ancient, most universal, most destructive which has become the mother of various (acute) and chronic (non-venereal) diseases. Origin of psora is related to spiritualism. It is spiritual sickness. Wrong thoughts and wrong desires give origin to psora and it makes him susceptible to all diseases.

Argument

Now I am analyzing an important part of the homeopathic concept. Hahnemann said,

> Psora is that most ancient, most universal, most misapprehended, chronic miasmatic disease which for many thousands of years has disfigured and tortured mankind and which during the last centuries has become the mother of all the thousands of incredibly various (acute and) chronic (non-venereal) diseases by which the whole civilized human race on the inhabitat globe is being more and more afflicted. (Hahnemann, 1999, p. 35)

Kent writes,

> Psora is the beginning of all physical sickness. Had psora never been established as a miasm upon the human race, the other two chronic diseases would have been impossible and susceptibility to acute diseases would have been impossible. All the diseases of man are built upon psora; hence it is the foundation of sickness. All other sickness came afterwards. (Kent, 1993, p. 126)

According to homeopathy, psora is a most important miasm and root of all the diseases. Now the important thing is to know about the origin

DOI: 10.1201/9781003228622-47

of psora. How did psora originate? Kent said that the origin of psora is related to spiritualism. When people went against the religion, psora originated. "If the human race had remained in a state of perfect order, psora could not have existed ... that is the spiritual sickness from which first states the race progressed into what may be called the true susceptibility to psora which in turn laid the foundation for other diseases" (Kent, 1993, p. 126).

Kent also explained,

> Thinking and willing establishes a state in man that identifies the condition he is in. As long as man continued to think that which was true and held that which was good to the neighbour, that which was uprightness and justice, so long man remained upon the earth free from the susceptibility to disease because that was the state in which he was created. So long as he remained in that state and preserved his integrity, he was not susceptible to disease and he gave forth no aura that could cause contagion but when man began to will the things that were the outcome of his false thinking then he entered a state which was the perfect correspondence of his interior. As the life of man or as the will of man so is the body of man. (Kent, 1993, p. 134)

Kent says that it is the wrong thought and wrong desires which give origin to psora and this psora makes him susceptible to all diseases. Environment cannot make him susceptible to diseases. Environment is not the cause of disease.

> The internal state of man is prior to that which surrounds him, therefore the environment is not the cause, it is only as if it were a sounding board. It only reacts upon and reflects the internal. One who has the prior, which is internal, may have that which can follow upon the external, it flows as it were from the internal and affects its forms upon the skin, upon the organs, upon the body of man. (Kent, 1993, p. 136)

Hahnemann also said that syphilis and sycosis were also complicated by coexistence of psora. In syphilis and sycosis, lesions were externally localized but after destruction of externally localized lesions, disease

Chapter forty seven: Psora and spiritualism 193

spread into internal organs due to the presence of psora. Hahnemann writes, "Syphilis and sycosis when complicated with developed psora, it is impossible to cure the venereal disease alone without treating psora" (Hahnemann, 1999, p. 163).

Various concepts were made by Hahnemann and Kent regarding the origin and development of psora. When we analyze these concepts in the context of present medical knowledge and find that conclusions drawn in homeopathy about psora were also inaccurate and false.

References

Hahnemann, S. (1999). *The chronic diseases (theoretical part)* (Reprint ed.) New Delhi, India: B Jain Publishers.

Kent, J. T. (1993). *Lectures on homeopathic philosophy.* Delhi, India: B. Jain Publishers.

chapter forty eight

St. Anthony's fire and leprosy

Basic concept of homeopathy – forty eight

God warned that he should be followed otherwise men will suffer from tuberculosis and fever. During evolution, psora was in the form of St. Anthony's fire; during the middle ages, it resumed the form of leprosy.

Argument

Homeopathy says, "During evolution psora was in the form of St. Anthony's fire, during the middle ages, resumed the form of leprosy" (Hahnemann, 1999, p. 37).

Hahnemann supported religion in the prevention of diseases. He took support of Moses who had said, "Bodily defects which must not be found in a priest who is to offer sacrifice" (Hahnemann, 1999, p. 36).

Kent also said, "Patients are so well instructed not to do anything, to take no drugs, to keep the life as pure as possible, to keep the physical forces untrammeled by violence" (Kent, 1993, p. 130). Kent writes,

> Hence this state, the state of human mind and the state of the human body, is a state of susceptibility to disease from willing evils, from thinking that which is false and making life one continuous heredity of false things and so this form of disease, psora, is but an outward manifestation of that which is prior in man. (Kent, 1993, p. 135)

"Leprosy prevails today up on the face of the earth but it prevails in a milder form in the form of psora. A new contagion comes with every child. As psora piles up generation after generation, century after century the susceptibility to it increases" (Kent, 1993, p. 135).

Hahnemann took the concept of the origin of psora from the Bible. It is mentioned in the Bible, "Whatever a man thinks, he thinks bad. God observed, evils have increased on the earth. Then God repented regarding the creation of men and decided to punish and abolish them" (The Holy Bible, creation, 6.5–6.8, p. 4). "God warned that he should be followed

DOI: 10.1201/9781003228622-48

otherwise men will suffer from tuberculosis and fever" (The Holy Bible, levy-vyavastha, 26.15–26.16, p. 73).

Kent mentioned

> Long before the time of Noah's flood, which was an inundation that destroyed the evil ones that were upon the earth at that time, there was a manifestation called leprosy which was but the result of the dreadful profanity that took place in this period. A great many people suffered then from the violent aura of leprosy whereas the natural disorder of the human race today is a milder form of psora upon a different race of people. If we had the same race upon the earth today we would have leprosy among them as we now have the milder form of psora. The ancients referred to leprosy as an internal itch. (Kent, 1993, p. 134)

Noah's flood is mentioned in the Bible. It has been said, "Noah was a religious person that's why he had been protected by god and other persons on earth were non religious and full of evils therefore they all were destroyed by flood" (The Holy Bible, creation, 7.6–7.24, p. 5).

Kent said that prior to Noah's flood, many people had suffered from the violent aura and leprosy and this leprosy was nothing but a form of psora. Hahnemann writes, "The occidental psora which during the middle ages, had raged in Europe for several centuries under the form of malignant erysipelas called St Anthony's Fire, resumed the form of leprosy" (Hahnemann, 1999, p. 37).

What is St. Anthony's fire? St. Anthony's fire was actually toxic manifestations of ergot poisoning.

> Ergot is a fungus to which rye is particularly susceptible ... The eating of bread made from contaminated rye was responsible in the past for many outbreaks of ergotism ... The effects of ergotism are alarming and explain why the disease was once regarded with superstitious dread. The most usual symptoms of ergotism was gangrene which was a consequence of vasoconstriction and which resulted in fingers, toes or whole limbs becoming dried, shrivelled and black so that they sometimes fell off ... It was for this reason (and perhaps also because the blackened limbs appeared to have

Chapter forty eight: St. Anthony's fire and leprosy

> been charred by fire) that ergotism was popularly known as St. Anthony's fire. St. Anthony's name was attached because it was believed that pilgrims to his shrine would be cured of this affliction. This promise did not go entirely unfulfilled for the act of pilgrimage ensured that the victim left the area in which the infected rye was growing. Ergotism is also associated with the occurrence of spontaneous abortions and with disturbance of central nervous function including convulsions and acute mania. (Crossland, 1980, p. 294)

The St. Anthony fire was misunderstood as a punishment of a non-religious act. But in fact it was toxic manifestations of ergot, a compound present in rye. This compound was not present in bread made in the shrine of St. Anthony because crops of this area were not contaminated with infected rye. When people remained in the shrine of St. Anthony, they must not have suffered from the St. Anthony fire.

Homeopathy is one of the best examples where lack of knowledge is responsible for the development of wrong therapeutic methods.

The first and the most important concept that is absolutely wrong is the concept of psora. Whatever Hahnemann said about psora is absolutely wrong. He said, "Psora originated due to wrong thought and psora was modified into St. Anthony Fire and leprosy. All diseases except syphilis and sycosis are due to psora".

Conclusion derived by Hahnemann after observation of leprosy patients was also wrong. In leprosy, "various clinical forms attack superficial tissues especially the skin, peripheral nerves and nasal mucosa" (Shepard, 1983, p. 1030). The rest of the body remains healthy. Hahnemann concluded, "This was owing to the obstinately persistent eruption on the skin, which served as a substitute for the internal psora" (Hahnemann, 1999, p. 38).

Hahnemann said the persistence of external eruption is a must to maintain health. He erroneously understood in leprosy that external symptomatic lesions are responsible for maintaining the health of leprosy patients and he made a wrong generalization of it. He committed this mistake due to a lack of knowledge.

> Even in the most advanced lepromatous cases destructive lesions are limited to the skin, peripheral nerves, anterior portion of the eye, upper respiratory passages above the larynx, testes, structures of the hands and feet. The probable reason for the

predilection of the disease for these tissues is that they are all usually several degrees cooler than 37°C … In mice that have been experimentally infected in the foot pads, bacillary multiplication is maximal when the mice are kept at air temperature at which the foot pad tissues are about 30°C; this is also the usual temperature of the most severely involved tissues of human beings. (Shepard, 1983, p. 1030)

"As one studying the lesions of leprosy clinically, it is evident that mycobacterium leprae, causative organism of leprosy appears to grow best in parts of the body that are relatively cool" (Binford, 1971, p. 338). In leprosy, destruction of comparatively cooler parts of the body is the characteristic feature. These are not the external symptoms that make the remaining body healthy. In this way so many wrong observations and generalizations were made by Hahnemann.

References

Binford, C. H. (1971). Leprosy. In W.A.D. Anderson (Ed.), *Pathology* (6th ed., Vol 1, pp. 328–340). St. Louis, MO: C.V. Mosby Company.

Crossland, J. (1980). *Lewis's pharmacology* (5th ed.). New York, NY: Churchill Livingstone.

Hahnemann, S. (1999). *The chronic diseases (theoretical part)* (Reprint ed.). New Delhi, India: B Jain Publishers.

Kent, J. T. (1993). *Lectures on homeopathic philosophy.* Delhi, India: B. Jain Publishers.

Shepard, C. C. (1983). Leprosy. In R. G. Petersdorf, R. D. Adams, E. Braunwald, K. J. Isselbacher, J. B. Martin, & J. D. Wilson (Eds.), *Harrison's principle of internal medicine* (10th ed., pp. 1030–1032). New Delhi, India: McGraw Hill.

Chapter forty nine

Pathogenesis of psora

Basic concept of homeopathy – forty nine

After the destruction of external skin eruptions, psora plays the sad role of causing innumerable secondary symptoms. When skin eruptions subside, severe manifestations are the result. Psora spreads from one person to another person. When internal development of psora has been completed, vital force develops skin eruption as a substitute for the internal psora and keeps the psora in a confined and stable position.

Argument

Hahnemann writes about causes of chronic diseases, "At the end of the fifteenth century, psora appeared only in the form of the common eruption of itch" (Hahnemann, 1999, p. 37). "In the last three centuries of its chief symptom, the external skin eruption, psora plays the sad role of causing innumerable secondary symptoms" (Hahnemann, 1999, p. 41).

> The psora which is now so easily and so rashly robbed of its ameliorating cutaneous symptom the eruption of itch, which acts vicariously for the internal disease, has been producing within the last three hundred years more and more secondary symptoms and indeed, so many that at least seven eights of all the chronic maladies spring from it as their only source while the remaining eighth springs from syphilis and sycosis. (Hahnemann, 1999, pp. 42–43)

All diseases except sexually transmitted diseases are due to psora, Hahnemann said. He did not mention how psora causes these all diseases. Neither he mentioned pathogenesis nor he mentioned different specific etiological agents. Hahnemann also did not describe features of psora and he also did not give any evidence except a hypothesis. He gave a list of diseases and said these all are due to hypothetical psora. He said,

> So great a flood of numberless nervous trouble, painful ailments, spasms, ulcers (cancers), adventitious

DOI: 10.1201/9781003228622-49

199

> formations, dyscrasias, paralysis, consumptions
> and crippling of soul, mind and body were never
> seen in ancient times when the psora mostly con-
> fined itself to its dreadful cutaneous symptoms
> leprosy. Only during the last few centuries has
> mankind been flooded with these infirmities owing
> to the causes just mentioned. It was thus the psora
> became the most universal mother of chronic dis-
> eases. (Hahnemann, 1999, p. 42)

List of symptoms given by Hahnemann caused by psora are ver-
tigo, dizziness, rush of blood to head, heat in the head, headache, roaring
noise in the brain, dandruff eruption on the head, tinea capitis, bald-
ness, paleness, redness of face, erysipelas, inflammation of eye, dropsy
of eye, cataract, squint, far sightedness, short sightedness, double vision,
night blindness, amaurosis, running pulsation and various sounds in
the ear, deafness, swelling of the parotid gland, epistaxis, polypi of the
nose, sense of smell perverted, redness and swelling of lips, gum disease,
toothache, looseness of teeth, coated tongue, inflammation and bitter test
in mouth, eructations, heart burn, water brash, nausea, vomiting, cough,
hiccough, ravenous hunger, appetite without hunger, spasm in stomach,
distension of abdomen, tired and sleepy, headache, after meals pain in
abdomen, colic, hardness of abdomen, uterine spasm, inguinal her-
nias, constipation, diarrhea, problems about stool, hemorrhoids, polypi
in the rectum, pain, full retention of urine, erosion in the anus and the
perineum, urine of different colors, diabetes, sexual problems, disappearance of testicles, impotency, sterility, enlargement of prostate gland,
menstrual disorder, polypi in the vagina, leucorrhea, coryza, laryngo
bronchial phthisis, aphony and hoarseness of voice, cough, whooping
cough, pain in chest, nightmare, asthma, suffocations, palpitations, excessive enlargement of breast, pain in the back, burning and itching in the
heal and soles, painful swollen joints, softening of bones, curvature of the
spine, fragility of bone, intolerable pain and numbness of the skin, varices,
whitlow, paronychia, chilblains, corns, boils, furuncle, ulcers; tumefaction
and suppuration of the humerus, the femur, patella, bone of fingers and
toes; eruptions, warts, encysted tumors in the skin and cellular tissue,
perspirations, faintness, tetanus, tremor, loss of consciousness, epilepsy,
insomnia, somnambulism, intermittent fever, disturbance of the mind
and spirit of all kinds, anxiety, mania, quick change of mood, disinclina-
tion to work (Hahnemann, 1999, pp. 105–143). Hahnemann said, "These
are the symptoms, observed by me which, if they are often repeated or
become constant, show the internal psora is coming forth from its latent
state" (Hahnemann, 1999, p. 143).

Chapter forty nine: Pathogenesis of psora 201

At the time of Hahnemann, there were no knowledge regarding etiological agents, pathogenesis, clinical symptomatology, clinical diagnosis, investigations, and natural prognosis of diseases, that's why Hahnemann presumed by mistake that all diseases are due to psora without giving specific name to diseases.

Every person suffers from one or some other health problem in his life. And this is also true that every person also suffers with some skin manifestations in his lifetime. Hahnemann correlated these two events and said every disease except sexually transmitted disease is due to psora which is represented in the body by external skin eruptions during latent state. Hahnemann also said by mistake that when skin eruptions subside severe manifestations result. He also said that psora spreads from one person to another.

Hahnemann writes,

> The itch disease is however also the most contagious of all chronic miasmata, far more infectious than the other two chronic miasmata the venereal chancre disease and the fig-wart disease. To affect the infection with the latter there is required a certain amount of friction in the most tender parts of the body which are the most rich in nerves and covered with the thinnest cuticle, as in the genital organs unless the miasma should touch a wounded spot. But the miasma of the itch needs only to touch the general skin especially with tender children. The disposition of being affected with the miasma of the itch is found with almost every one and under almost all circumstances, which is not the case with the other two miasmata. (Hahnemann, 1999, pp. 78–79)

When psora spreads from one person to another person then what happens? Hahnemann writes,

> As soon as the miasma of itch e.g. touches the hand, in the moment when it has taken effect, it no more remains local. Henceforth all washing and cleansing of the spot avails nothing. Nothing is seen on the skin during the first days, it remains unchanged and according to appearance, healthy … Living organism, has at once, all unperceived, been so penetrated by this specific excitation … until the change

202   *Homeopathy*

of the whole being to a man thoroughly psoric and thus the internal development of the psora has reached completion. (Hahnemann, 1999, p. 80)

When internal development of psora has been completed then what will be the position of health? Body is diseased or the body remains healthy. Hahnemann says,

> Only when the whole organism feels itself transformed by this peculiar chronic miasmatic disease, the diseased vital force endeavors to alleviate and to soothe the internal malady through the establishment of a suitable local symptom on the skin, the itch vesicles. So long as this eruption continues in its normal form the internal psora, with its secondary ailments cannot break forth but must remain covered, slumbering, latent and bound. (Hahnemann, 1999, p. 81)

These eruption symptoms work as a substitute for the internal malady and keep the psora in a confined and stable position.

Hahnemann also said herpes and tinea capitis were representations of internal psora. "These alone can propagate this disease to other persons because they alone contain the communicable miasm of psora" (Hahnemann, 1999, p. 82). Hahnemann did not know the fact that herpes is a viral infection and tinea capitis is a fungal infection. He thought that both are different manifestations of psora.

Reference

Hahnemann, S. (1999). *The chronic diseases* (theoretical part) (Reprint ed.). New Delhi, India: B Jain Publishers.

chapter fifty

Awakening of internal psora

Basic concept of homeopathy – fifty

Slumbering and bound psora awake and outbreak due to improper treatment by allopathic physician through some unlucky physical or psychical occurrence, a violent fright, continual vexations, deeply affecting grief, catching a severe cold, or a cold temperature, etc. Suppression of itch is mainly responsible for awakening of internal psora that gives many chronic symptomatology and diseases.

Argument

Now there is a question, how does this slumbering and bound psora awake and outbreak? Hahnemann answers this question. Hahnemann says, "Most of all through weakening and exhausting improper treatment by allopathic physicians" (Hahnemann, 1999, p. 98). The other causes of awakening of psora as mentioned by Hahnemann are

> The eruption of itch by no means remains as persistently in its place on the skin as the chancre and figwart. Even if the eruption of itch has not (as is nearly always the case) been driven away from the skin through the faulty practice of physicians and quacks by means of desiccating washes, sulfur ointments, drastic purgatives or cupping. It frequently disappears as we say of itself i.e. through causes which are not noticed. It often, disappears through some unlucky physical or physical occurrence through a violent fright, through continual vexations, deeply affecting grief, through catching a severe cold or through a cold temperature, through cold, lukewarm and warm river baths or mineral bath, by a fever arising from any cause or through a different acute disease ... through persistent diarrhoea, sometimes also perhaps through a peculiar want of activity in the skin, and the results in such a case are just as mischievous as if the eruption had been

DOI: 10.1201/9781003228622-50

driven away externally by the irrational practice of a physician. The secondary ailments of the internal psora and any one of the innumerable chronic diseases flowing from this origin will then break out sooner or later. (Hahnemann, 1999, pp. 40–41)

Suppression of itch is mainly responsible for the awakening of internal psora that gives many chronic symptomatology and diseases.

The main concept of homeopathy regarding psora and chronic diseases is suppression of itch. Hahnemann said,

Psora manifests itself when the external local symptoms which serve to assuage the internal malady is hastily removed ... The diseases partly acute but chiefly chronic springing from such a one sided destruction of the chief skin symptoms (eruptions and itching) which acts vicariously and assuage the internal psora. (Hahnemann, 1999, pp. 47–48)

Hahnemann said again and again that all chronic diseases are due to suppression of eruption and itch. When asked how suppression of itch transformed into diseases, he said nothing. What are the characteristic features of psora, he again said nothing.

Hahnemann quoted the observation of Ludwig Christian Juncker in support of suppression of itch and origin of diseases.

He observed that with young people of a sanguine temperament, the suppression of itch is followed by phthisis and with persons in general who are of a sanguine temperament, it is followed by piles, haemorrhoidal colic and renal gravels; with persons of sanguine choleric temperament by swelling of the inguinal glands, stiffening of the joints and malignant ulcers; with fat persons by a suffocating catarrh and mucous consumption also by inflammatory fever, acute pleurisy and inflammation of lung ... Phlegmatic persons in consequence of such suppressions suffered chiefly from dropsy, menses were delayed and when the itch was driven away during their flow they were changed into a monthly hemoptysis. Persons inclined to melancholy were sometimes made insane by such repression, if they were pregnant the foetus was usually killed.

Chapter fifty: *Awakening of internal psora*

Sometimes the suppression of itch causes sterility.
(Hahnemann, 1999, pp. 48–49)

Now it is clear that in homeopathy, bad thinking leads to the origin of psora, which "for many thousands of years had disfigured and tortured mankind and which during the last centuries has become the mother of all the thousands of incredibly various (acute) and chronic (non-venereal) diseases" (Hahnemann, 1999, p. 35).

Reference

Hahnemann, S. (1999). *The chronic diseases (theoretical part)* (Reprint ed.). New Delhi, India: B Jain Publishers.

chapter fifty one

Suppression of itch and tinea capitis

Basic concept of homeopathy – fifty one

Hahnemann presented a list of 97 examples of different clinical manifestations and proved by simple observation of appearance and disappearance of lesions that all clinical problems were due to suppression of itch. There are 15 examples in the list where suppression of tinea complex results in secondary diseases.

Argument

Now I will explain how Hahnemann reached the wrong conclusion of suppression of itch and the origin of diseases. At that time, there was no knowledge regarding etiology and pathogenesis of diseases. According to his own knowledge and imagination, the hypothesis was established without experimental studies. Hahnemann said, "The causes of all diseases are psora, syphilis and sycosis. Psora is the mother of all diseases". It was the imagination of Hahnemann. Most of the cases of syphilis and sycosis were cured spontaneously. Hahnemann thought that he was curing the diseases by only a single dose of drug with dilutions up to 10^{60}. As I have already written, many diseases are cured spontaneously; that's why different pathies get a false reputation as an effective therapy. Homeopathy also got such a false reputation and became popular.

Hahnemann developed the concept of psora for non-venereal diseases. Spontaneous cure of syphilis and sycosis gave false confidence to Hahnemann regarding his work. The concept of psora was based on wrong conclusions, which were derived by observing one or two cases of different diseases. Hahnemann never did controlled study in patients. He made a very simple statement that the presence of psora in the body is represented by itch or skin eruptions and suppression of itch is responsible for secondary manifestations of many chronic diseases.

Medical facts cannot be derived on the basis of only one or two examples. This mistake was committed by Hahnemann and his followers.

DOI: 10.1201/9781003228622-51

Hahnemann writes that eruption of itch also disappears through catching a severe cold, a cold temperature, or vexation or grief (Hahnemann, 1999, p. 41). In support of this conclusion, he instructed us to see observation no. 67. In this observation, "A man whose tinea capitis had passed off from intense cold was seized after eight days with a malignant fever with vomiting accompanied at last with hiccough. He died in consequence on the 9th day" (Hahnemann, 1999, p. 62).

Hahnemann presented a list of 97 examples of different clinical manifestations and proved by simple observation of appearance and disappearance of lesions that all clinical problems were due to suppression of itch. In example 5, it is mentioned,

> A boy of 13 years having suffered from his childhood with tinea capitis, had his mother removed it for him but he became very sick within 8 or 10 days, suffering with asthma, violent pain in the limbs, back and knee which were not relieved until an eruption of itch broke out over his whole body a month later. (Hahnemann, 1999, p. 51)

There are 25 examples in the list, where suppression of tinea capitis infection results in secondary clinical manifestations. In example 5, suppression of tinea capitis results in asthma. In example 6, tinea capitis was driven away by purgative and produced symptoms of cough and lassitude. In example 16, suppression of tinea capitis produced fever, and in other examples suppression of tinea is responsible for blood in skull, putrefied brain, swelling of the glands of neck, violent fever, pain in back, and headache (Hahnemann, 1999).

Hahnemann says that tinea capitis is not a localized disease. He also says, "Localized disease is not possible. According to him all localized lesions are external manifestations of generalized disease. Without general involvement local lesions are not possible". But Hahnemann was wrong, it can be explained very well. Tinea infection is a fungus infection and it is localized without general involvement. Scabies, boils, carbuncle, contact dermatitis, pityriasis versicolor, and localized candida infection. Skin carcinomas are also localized lesions.

Tinea capitis is a chronic fungal infection. Acquisition of a fungal infection (dermatophyte) appears to be favored by minor trauma, maceration, and poor hygiene of the skin. Usually dermatophytes infections are cured spontaneously due to the reason given here.

> Invasion of the stratum corneum by dermatophytes (ringworm or tinea) may cause little inflammation or

Chapter fifty one: Suppression of itch and tinea capitis 209

> particularly with zoophilic fungi inflammation can be intense. Shedding of the stratum corneum is increased by inflammation, to the extent that fungal growth cannot keep up with shedding. Inflammation may help terminate infection. Conversely infection is probably favoured when shedding is reduced by corticosteroids and cytotoxic drugs. (Bennett, 1983, p. 1065)

Today through knowledge of scientific medical study, we know that suppression of tinea capitis can never produce any other disease. Asthma, fever, and pain can never be produced by the suppression of tinea. It was the wrong observation by Hahnemann. Neither suppression of tinea was related to the development of asthma, fever, or other manifestations nor reappearance of tinea infection was related to the cure of these diseases. It was just the coexistence of two different diseases and nothing else.

In the list of observations, Hahnemann quoted 13 examples of asthma (Hahnemann, 1999, pp. 49–69). He concluded that suppression of tinea/rash/itch resulted in asthma and reappearance of skin lesions again resulted in recovery. If skin lesions are not appeared again, then there is a possibility of death from asthma as mentioned in example 15, 69 and 70. Facts about asthma were not known to Hahnemann. He was thinking that asthma was due to the suppression of itch, rash, or tinea and reappearance of rash, itch, or tinea resulted in cure. But facts are as follows,

> Asthma is manifested physiologically by a widespread narrowing of the air passage which may be relieved spontaneously or as a result of therapy. Asthma is manifested clinically by paroxysms of dyspnoea, cough and wheezing. It is an episodic disease, acute exacerbations being interspersed with symptom free periods. Typically most attacks are short lived lasting minutes to hours and after them the patient seems to recover completely clinically. (McFadden & Austen, 1983, p. 1512)

> Allergic asthma is frequently seasonal and it is most often observed in children and young adults. Allergic asthma is ... The history of periodic attacks are quite characteristic. A personal or family history of allergic diseases such as eczema, rhinitis,

urticaria is valuable contributory evidence ... The natural course of asthma in adult life has been little investigated. Some studies suggest that spontaneous remissions occur in approximately 20 percent of those who develop the disease as adults and 40% or so can be expected to improve with less frequent and severe attacks as they grow older. (McFadden & Austen, 1983, pp. 1512–1519)

Now it is clear that asthma of the allergic type is usually associated with eczema or urticaria that is skin lesion. In other words, skin lesions are usually associated with allergic asthma. Suppression of skin lesions never produces asthma. Another interesting finding of asthma is

It is paroxysmal. A person who is subject to asthma may be perfectly well one minute and half an hour later may be in the throes of a violent attack. An attack may last minutes, hours or days and when prolonged is termed status asthmaticus. As the attack subsides, breathing becomes gradually easier, the patient often coughs up a plug of mucus sputum and then rapidly recovers. There are many interesting features in this disease such as a personal history of skin eruptions (urticaria, prurigo and eczema), these often alternating with paroxysms of asthma. (Warner, 1964, p. 211)

Regarding prognosis, "Children frequently grow out of the disease about puberty. Adults never lose the tendency to attack but may be free for years" (Warner, 1964, p. 214).

Now we summarize total characteristic features of asthma.
Paroxysmal episodic character.
Free intervals of varying periods between attacks.
Associated with skin lesions.
Skin eruptions are present often alternating with paroxysms of asthma.
Chances of spontaneous recovery.
Children frequently grow out of the disease about puberty.

On the basis of the above conclusions, it can be said that Hahnemann's views about the origin and cure of asthma were wrong. The origin and recovery from asthma are not due to appearance or suppression of eruptions.

Chapter fifty one: Suppression of itch and tinea capitis 211

References

Bennett, J. E. (1983). Dermatophytosis. In R. G. Petersdorf, R. D. Adams, E. Braunwald, K. J. Isselbacher, J. B. Martin, & J. D. Wilson (Eds.), *Harrison's principle of internal medicine* (10th ed., pp. 1065–1066). New Delhi, India: McGraw Hill.

Hahnemann, S. (1999). *The chronic diseases (theoretical part)* (Reprint ed.). New Delhi, India: B Jain Publishers.

McFadden, E. R., Jr, & Austen, K. F. (1983). Dermatophytosis. In R. G. Petersdorf, R. D. Adams, E. Braunwald, K. J. Isselbacher, J. B. Martin, & J. D. Wilson (Eds.), *Harrison's principle of internal medicine* (10th ed., pp. 1512–1519). New Delhi, India: McGraw Hill.

Warner, E. C. (Ed). (1964). *Savill's system of clinical medicine* (14th ed.). London, United Kingdom: Edward Arnold Publisher.

chapter fifty two

Epilepsy and exanthema

Basic concept of homeopathy – fifty two

Time interval is different in different cases after suppression of itch and development of secondary disease. Epilepsy and fever are also developed due to suppression of itch. Reappearance of itch and eruption is a must for cure.

Argument

Hahnemann did not give any explanation of how suppression of rash creates disease. He also did not explain how only one mechanism that is suppression of itch developed different diseases in different persons. He did not tell how much time will be taken in the development of secondary manifestations after suppression of itch. In example 75, he quoted,

> A count, 57 years old, had suffered for three years with dry itch. It was driven off and he enjoyed for two years apparently good health, only he had during this time two attacks of vertigo.... A similar attack followed six weeks later than once a month for three months. (Hahnemann, 1999, p. 64)

In example 81, it is written, "A youth of 18 years drove off the itch with a mercurial ointment and two months after he was unexpectedly seized with convulsions" (Hahnemann, 1999, p. 66). In example 85, It is mentioned, "A youth of 18, who had driven out itch with mercurial remedies was seized a few weeks later with epilepsy, which returned after four weeks with the new moon" (Hahnemann, 1999, p. 66). In example 88, it is mentioned, "Five year old itch passed away and this after several years produced epilepsy" (Hahnemann, 1999, p. 67).

In examples 75, 85, and 88, time intervals are different in different cases after suppression of itch and development of secondary manifestations. In example 75, it is two years; in example 81, it is two months; in example 85, it is a few weeks; and in example 88, it is several years. In these examples, in one case, epilepsy is produced two months after suppression of itch; in other cases, epilepsy is produced after a few weeks

DOI: 10.1201/9781003228622-52

214   *Homeopathy*

and after several years of suppression of itch. In many cases, secondary manifestations are developed soon after suppression of itch. This shows that this correlation is not accurate. In the list of 97 examples, 11 are of epilepsy. It has been also said about epilepsy that this was originated due to suppression of itch. It is not true. Hahnemann should have thought about how, in one case, epilepsy developed soon after suppression of itch and, in another case, epilepsy developed after many years of suppression of itch. But he did not analyze accurately. Skin eruptions, itch, skin lesions, boil, acne, eczema, fungal infection, and many other skin diseases are very common. Everybody suffers from one or other localized skin diseases sometimes in his life. He also suffers from many other diseases. Hahnemann falsely correlated both these.

Epilepsy is a group of disorders characterized by chronic recurrent paroxysmal changes in neurological function caused by abnormal electrical activity of the brain. Causes of seizures are intracranial birth injury, acute infection, metabolic disturbances, genetic disorders, febrile convulsion, alcoholism, brain tumor, and cardiovascular disease (Dichter, 1983, pp. 2018–2027). "Epileptic attacks usually recur at intervals throughout life but in some cases they disappear spontaneously either for years or permanently. Occasionally isolated fits may not be repeated" (Warner, 1964, p. 1141).

> Convulsions in infancy are not necessarily followed by epilepsy in adult life. Pyknolepsy (attacks of minor epilepsy in children) is said to disappear completely at puberty. In some cases one or two fits occur in adolescence and then a long remission follows. In exceptional cases, isolated major fits may occur in adult life and not recur. Most confirmed epileptics are able to live a normal working life under selected conditions away from potential danger (machinery, furnaces, heights) and to many have healthy children. (Warner, 1964, p. 1147)

We have seen that causes of epilepsy are not related to skin lesions and attacks of epilepsy are recurrent. Time interval is not fixed for recurrent attacks. Attacks may recur on the same day or a second attack may come after a gap of months or years. There is also a possibility that epilepsy may not recur at all. Then this statement that epilepsy occurs due to suppression of itch is absolutely wrong.

At present, there is no evidence that localized treatment of skin disease causes the development of secondary diseases. If Hahnemann is right, then all skin specialists should be banned. There should not be provision

Chapter fifty two: Epilepsy and exanthema 215

of skin specialists according to homeopathy, because they mainly suppress or treat localized skin lesions externally. Homeopathy says, "Skin specialists are dangerous. They create many severe secondary diseases by removing localized skin lesions". Do you agree with this pseudo fact? Should skin specialists be banned?

There were 16 cases of fever and associated symptoms in this list. It had been said by Hahnemann that fever was due to suppression of itch and reappearance of itch or eruption is a must for cure of fever, as written in example 72, "After driving off itch, most frequently acute fevers with a great sinking of the strength follows. In one such case the fever lasted seven days, when the eruption of itch reappeared and stopped the fever" (Hahnemann, 1999, p. 63).

There are many diseases of fever where skin eruptions appear. But suppression of eruptions is not the cause of disease and reappearance of eruptions is not the cause of cure. Many fevers have eruptions as a sign of disease. Eruptions are manifestations of diseases and appearance and disappearance are related to the stage of disease. Examples of such disease are (1) viral infection: rubeola, rubella, hepatitis, measles, arboviruses, adenoviruses, vaccinia, herpes simplex, dengue, and yellow fever; (2) bacterial infection: scarlet fever, erysipelas, subacute bacterial endocarditis, typhoid fever, bullous, impetigo, gonococcemia, and *Haemophilus influenzae*; (3) rickettsial: rocky mountain spotted fever and epidemic typhus; (4) fungal: candidiasis and sporotrichosis; (5) chlamydial psittacosis; (6) protozoal: toxoplasmosis and trichinosis; (7) immunological ; and (8) drug eruptions.

> The pathogenesis of an exanthem may be caused by (1) Multiplication of the pathogen in the skin. (2) Carriage of the agent in plasma or in infected hematopoietic cells (leukocytes and or lymphocytes) into integumentary blood vessels (3) Antigen antibody or delayed hypersensitivity reactions to antigen derived from the infecting microorganisms ... Regional multiplication of the virus, primary viremia and visceral dissemination of virus occur prior to the development of the exanthem and explain why the initial clinical manifestations of many viral illnesses occur prior to the development of the rash ... In some petechial eruptions direct evidence of viral or bacterial invasion can be obtained by direct aspiration and culture of the lesion, by demonstrating the agent with Gram's stain or by immunofluorescent stain to detect microbial agents. (Corex, 1983, p. 1109)

216 *Homeopathy*

> Some exanthematous diseases produce characteristic cutaneous patterns ... Streptococcus produces a rash that starts on the neck and spreads to the trunk and extremities within 36 hours ... The course of the eruption is also helpful in differentiating the etiology of viral exanthems ... The eruption of rubella tends to disappear from its original site of involvement as it spreads ... The cutaneous lesions tend to wax and wane with fever. (Corex, 1983, pp. 1109–1111)

"In each acute exanthemata, the eruption has a special and distinctive character, which together with the day of the disease on which the eruption appears may enable one to differentiate the members of this group from one another" (Warner, 1964, p. 669).

In chicken pox, rash appears on the first day of pyrexia; in scarlet fever, it appears on the second day; in smallpox, it appears on the third day; and in measles, rash appears on the fourth day of pyrexia (Warner, 1964, p. 669).

Rash appears and disappears according to disease present. In chicken pox, within 24 hours, the characteristic eruptions appear; after a few days, lesion dries into a scab that within 10–14 days separates, leaving a pigmented area (Warner, 1964, p. 670). In scarlet fever, "The rash continues to be well marked until the fourth or fifth day of the disease but disappears earlier if antitoxin or penicillin have been given ... the rash indicates the production of an erythrogenic toxin by the infecting organism" (Warner, 1964, pp. 673–674). "In erysipelas the rash may vary in duration from 3 to 4 days to a fortnight; it is materially shortened by chemotherapy" (Warner, 1964, p. 678).

> Dengue or break bone fever is a specific fever lasting not more than 7 days and mainly confined to tropical climates ... Often within 1 to 2 days the skin over the face, neck and chest becomes flushed and reddened (primary rash) ... by the 3rd or 4th day, the temperature falls to 100°F or lower, with sweating and perhaps diarrhoea. The patient temporarily feels better, but after a few hours to 3 days the temperature again rises ... the pain returns and a secondary rash appears which ... lasts a few hours to 3 days. Desquamation and itching follow. (Warner, 1964, p. 695)

Chapter fifty two: Epilepsy and exanthema 217

"In influenza eruptions of erythematous or urticarial type occur" (Warner, 1964, p. 702).

> In typhoid the rash generally appears about the seventh to twelfth day (average 10th) in successive crops of small rose coloured lenticular spots slightly elevated, soft and disappearing on pressure. Each spot lasts about 3 or 4 days; they are never petechial. They are chiefly seen on the abdomen. (Warner, 1964, p. 709)

By the above description, it should be clear that skin eruptions are a characteristic feature of diseases. Eruptions develop during pathogenesis of disease. Eruptions are parts of disease. Disease first enters the body, then eruption develops. Suppression of eruptions does not develop disease. Appearance of an eruption is not related to the cure of disease.

There are various other types of fevers where rash is not present. Examples are mumps, diphtheria, rheumatic fever, yellow fever, cat scratch fever, malaria, and amebiasis. These fevers are not related to rash. Then there is no question of establishing a relation between suppression of itch and origin of disease.

References

Corex, L. (1983). Approach to the patient with rash and fever. In R. G. Petersdorf, R. D. Adams, E. Braunwald, K. J. Isselbacher, J. B. Martin, & J. D. Wilson (Eds.), *Harrison's principle of internal medicine* (10th ed., pp. 1109–1113). New Delhi, India: McGraw Hill.

Dichter, M. A. (1983). The epilepsies and convulsive disorders. In R. G. Petersdorf, R. D. Adams, E. Braunwald, K. J. Isselbacher, J. B. Martin, & J. D. Wilson (Eds.), *Harrison's principle of internal medicine* (10th ed., pp. 2018–2028). New Delhi, India: McGraw Hill.

Hahnemann, S. (1999). *The chronic diseases (theoretical part)* (Reprint ed.). New Delhi, India: B Jain Publishers.

Warner, E. C. (Ed.). (1964). *Savill's system of clinical medicine* (14th ed.). London, United Kingdom: Edward Arnold Publisher.

chapter fifty three

Confusion

Basic concept of homeopathy – fifty three

Hahnemann himself quoted examples where without applying external allopathic treatment, eruptions were suppressed and created secondary clinical symptoms.

Argument

Hahnemann said repeatedly that suppression of external lesions or eruptions by external allopathic treatment is very dangerous and responsible for various secondary manifestations. "Hahnemann experiences were frequently confirmed by the observation of others" (Hahnemann, 1999, p. 49). Surprisingly, he himself quoted examples where without applying external ointment, eruptions were suppressed and created secondary symptoms, as written in case 64, "with a boy the itch passed away of itself, this was followed by fever" (Hahnemann, 1999, p. 62). In case 65, "Itch disappeared from the skin of itself, on which lingering fever, expectoration of pus and lastly death followed" (Hahnemann, 1999, p. 62).

In example 78, it is written, "A girl of 17 in consequence of Tinea capitis which disappeared of itself was seized with continuous heat in the head and attacks of headache" (Hahnemann, 1999, p. 65). External eruptions also passed off from cold as mentioned in case 67. "A man whose Tinea capitis had passed off from an intense cold was seized after eight days with a malignant fever with vomiting" (Hahnemann, 1999, p. 62).

Hahnemann emphasized mainly on removal of eruptions, fig wart, and chancre by allopathic doctors externally and said this is a very dangerous procedure, because these suppressed eruptions and suppressed external skin lesions cause widespread secondary manifestations. The same phenomenon also occurs itself as mentioned by Hahnemann in quoted examples. When we compare both these events, we find in one group secondary manifestations were present after applying external ointment, and in the second group, secondary manifestations were also present without applying external ointment. By this comparison, we can say that the development of secondary manifestations is not related to the application of external ointment. Again, we can say the hypothesis

DOI: 10.1201/9781003228622-53

219

and the conclusion of Hahnemann were wrong, and thus homeopathy was wrong.

These 97 examples were also the basis of the concept of psora. Hahnemann repeatedly quoted these examples for various conclusions. (1) In one example 91, a woman after having the itch driven out had paralysis of one leg; (2) in example 92, after driving off the itch with sulfur ointment, a man of 53 years had hemiplegia; (3) in example 47, driven off the itch with ointment leads to complicated kidney problem; (4) in example 27, after using ointment, patient passed away with anxiety, dyspnea, tenesmus, and the whole of lung was filled with liquid pus; (5) in example 30, diaphragm and the liver were diseased after using ointment; (6) in example 34, a boy of 7 weeks and a youth of 18 years died very suddenly from an itch driven out through a sulfur ointment; (7) in example 42, a vigorous man, when the itch had been expelled from the skin, was seized with amaurosis and remained blind to an advanced age; and (8) a man rubbed himself with mercurial ointment against the itch, when there followed an erysipelatous inflammation in the neck, of which he died after five weeks (Hahnemann, 1999, pp. 51–69).

As mentioned in the above references, according to Hahnemann, suppression of itch by itself or application of external ointment are mainly responsible for secondary manifestations. Hahnemann did not give any mechanism on how suppression leads to secondary diseases. He also did not explain which patient would suffer with what type of ailments after the suppression of eruptions. He also did not do controlled experiments.

Reference

Hahnemann, S. (1999). *The chronic diseases (theoretical part)* (Reprint ed.). New Delhi, India: B Jain Publishers.

chapter fifty four

Repetition of dose and medicine

Basic concept of homeopathy – fifty four

Homeopathy says that a single dose of homeopathic drug is effective orally and sufficient for complete cure in chronic diseases. New medicine and doses of the same medicine would interrupt the work of improvement and cause new ailments that often cannot be repaired for a long time. If somebody does this, he is unworthy of a homeopathic physician. In exceptional cases, repetition of dose is allowed but in different potencies. Homeopathic drugs are effective also by respiratory route. When treatment of infants is concerned, Hahnemann advised drug administration to nursing mothers.

Argument

Hahnemann writes regarding frequency of doses, "The disease of it being not one of very long standing will generally be removed and extinguished by the first dose of it without any considerable disturbance" (Hahnemann, 1921/1993, p. 218). He also writes,

> Every perceptible progressive and strikingly increasing amelioration during treatment is a condition which as long as it lasts completely precludes every repetition of the administration of any medicine ... in more chronic disease, on the other hand, a single dose of an appropriate selected homeopathic remedy will at time complete even with but slowly progressive improvement and give the help which such a remedy in such a case can accomplish naturally within 40, 50, 60, 100 days. (Hahnemann, 1921/2017, p. 205)

"It is impractical to repeat the same unchanged dose of a remedy once, not to mention its frequent repetition. The vital principle does not accept such an unchanged dose without resistance" (Hahnemann, 1921/1993, p. 272).

> The physician must therefore in chronic diseases allow all antipsoric remedies to act thirty, forty or

DOI: 10.1201/9781003228622-54

even fifty and more days by themselves, so long as they continue to improve the diseased state perceptibly to the acute observer, even though gradually, for so long the good effects continue with the indicated doses these must not be disturbed and checked by any new remedy. (Hahnemann, 1999, p. 212)

Why did Hahnemann oppose repetition of the same dose of medicine? He said,

A second dynamically wholly similar unchanged dose of the same medicine no longer finds, therefore the same condition of the vital force. The patient may indeed be made sick in another way by receiving other such unchanged doses, even sicker than he was, for now only those symptoms of the given remedy remain active which were not homeopathic to the original disease, hence no step towards cure can follow, only a true aggravation of the condition of the patient. (Hahnemann, 1921/2017, p. 206)

Hahnemann made a fundamental rule in the treatment of chronic diseases.

To let the action of the remedy selected in a mode homeopathic appropriate to the case of disease which has been carefully investigated to its symptoms, come to an undisturbed conclusion, so long as it visibly advances the cure and the while improvement still perceptibly progresses. This method forbids any new prescription, any interruption by another medicine and forbids as well immediate repetition of the same remedy. (Hahnemann, 1999, p. 214)

He said that new medicine and dose of the same medicine would interrupt the work of improvement and cause new ailments that often cannot be repaired for a long time. He writes, "Still there has been of late much abuse of this immediate repetition of doses of the same medicine, because young homeopaths thought it more convenient to repeat, without examination, a medicine which in the beginning had been found to be homeopathically suitable" (Hahnemann, 1999, p. 215).

We may declare at once, that the practice of late which has even been recommended in public

Chapter fifty four: Repetition of dose and medicine

journals, of giving the patient several doses of the same medicine to take with him, so that he may take them himself at certain intervals, without considering whether this repetition may affect him injuriously seems to show a negligent empiricism and to be unworthy of a homeopathic physician, who should not allow a new dose of a medicine to be taken or given without convincing himself in every case before hand as to its usefulness. (Hahnemann, 1999, p. 216)

Hahnemann advised,

The only allowable exception for an immediate repetition of the same medicine is when the dose of a well selected and in every way suitable and beneficial remedy has made some beginning toward an improvement, but its action ceases too quickly, its power is too soon exhausted and the cure does not proceed any further. This is rare in chronic diseases but in acute diseases and in chronic diseases that rise into an acute state, it is frequently the case … but this repetition should be permitted only when the preceding dose has largely exhausted its action (after six, eight or ten days) and the dose should be just as small as the preceding one and be given in a different potency. (Hahnemann, 1999, pp. 216–217)

Homeopathy says, a single dose of homeopathic drug is effective orally and sufficient for complete cure in chronic diseases. These drugs are also effective when taken through the respiratory route.

If only a small vial say a dram of dilute alcohol is used in the treatment, in which is contained and dissolved through succussion one globule of the medicine which is to be used by olfaction every two, three or four days, this also must be thoroughly succussed eight to ten times before each olfaction. (Hahnemann, 1921/1993, p. 275)

By such an inhalation the power of any potentized medicine may be communicated to the patient in any degree of strength … such medicated pellets kept in a stoppered vial retain their medicinal power quite undiminished, even if the vial be opened a number of times in many years for the purpose of inhalation; i.e., if the vial be preserved from sunshine and heat. (Hahnemann, 1999, p. 220)

Even persons born without the sense of smell or who have lost it through disease, may expect equally efficient help from drawing in the imperceptible vapor (proceeding from the medicine and contained in the vial) through one nostril or the other, as those who are gifted the sense of smell. From this it follows that the nerves possessing merely the sense touch receive the salutary impression and communicate unfailingly to the whole nervous system. (Hahnemann, 1999, pp. 219–220)

When treatment of infants is concerned, Hahnemann advised drug administration to the nursing mother. He said,

The power of medicines acting upon the infant through the milk of the mother of a wet nurse is wonderfully helpful. Every disease in a child yields to the rightly chosen homoeopathic medicines given in moderate doses to the nursing mother and so administered, is more easily and certainly utilized by these new world citizens than is possible in later years. Since most infants usually have imparted to them psora through the milk of the nurse, if they do not already possess it through heredity from the mother they may be at the same time protected antipsorically by means of the milk of the nurse rendered medicinally in this manner. (Hahnemann, 1921/2017, p. 234)

Hahnemann said, "Single dose of homeopathic drugs is sufficient in chronic diseases". There is no necessity for repetition of the drug. Effect lasts up to 50 or more days. In acute diseases, drugs can be repeated only in different potencies. The same drug with similar potency should not be repeated in homeopathy. If such a drug is repeated, then the drug will be harmful. For this conclusion, there is no experimental study in homeopathy. At present, homeopaths themselves do not follow this rule of Hahnemann. They use drugs in frequent doses with similar potency

Chapter fifty four: Repetition of dose and medicine 225

as they desire without any logic. Followers of homeopathy themselves are against the rules of Hahnemann.

See the statement of Hahnemann, which is highly ridiculous, illogical, and irrelevant. He says at one place for the treatment of infants, and drugs should be given to nursing mothers. Actually, what happened in spontaneously curable self-limiting diseases, whatever methods applied by Hahnemann, he thought that he had been able to treat the diseases successfully. In this way, he made the wrong concept of homeopathy.

References

Hahnemann, S. (1993). *Organon of medicine* (6th ed.) (W. Boericke, Trans.). New Delhi, India: B. Jain Publishers. (Original work published in 1921).

Hahnemann, S. (1999). *The chronic diseases (theoretical part)* (Reprint ed.). New Delhi, India: B Jain Publishers.

Hahnemann, S. (2017). *Organon of medicine* (6th ed.) (W. Boericke, Trans.). New Delhi, India: B. Jain Publishers. (Original work published in 1921).

chapter fifty five

Hahnemann accepted failure

Basic concept of homeopathy – fifty five

Hahnemann accepted failure of homeopathic treatment. He said that he was not able to cure all chronic patients. He mentioned many factors that made patients incurable and augmented their diseases.

Argument

Hahnemann got curative results in syphilis and sycosis by a homeopathic method of treatment because these diseases were cured spontaneously. He was convinced wrongly that he had been curing these patients. For the remaining diseases, he made another group of psora and he observed many case histories of patients and applied homeopathic law of treatment without doing controlled experiments.

Fatal diseases are those diseases where death is certain, if not properly treated. There is no possibility of spontaneous recovery in fatal disease. All patients with fatal diseases will definitely die if treatment is not available. AIDS, acquired immunodeficiency syndrome, is a fatal illness caused by a retrovirus. Rabies, also known as hydrophobia, is an acute highly fatal viral disease. These are two communicable diseases of man that are always fatal. Tropical diseases like malaria, fevers, typhoid, cholera, dysentery, amoebiasis, measles, chicken pox are not fatal diseases. In the absence of proper treatment, patients may die or recover spontaneously.

A maximum number of patients with tropical diseases, if not treated, recover spontaneously due to immunity in the body. Only a few patients die if not effectively treated. Without effective treatment, recovery may take longer time e.g., typhoid is cured spontaneously within a month in the absence of treatment but the presence of effective treatment cures typhoid within a week. "Without effective antibiotic treatment typhoid fever kills almost 10 percent of those infected" (Park, 1997, p. 174).

Case fatality rate represents the killing power of a disease. It is simply the ratio of deaths to cases. The time interval is not specified. The case fatality rate for the same disease may vary in different epidemics because of changes in the agent, host, and environmental factors. Case fatality is closely related to virulence.

DOI: 10.1201/9781003228622-55

228 *Homeopathy*

"Measles is a viral infection. In developing countries, case fatality rates range from 2 to 15 percent" (Park, 1997, p. 118). This indicates 2–15 deaths per 100 patients without treatment in measles. "In typhoid, case mortality varies in different epidemics from 5 to 20 percent" (Warner, 1964, p. 712). "Hepatitis B is a systemic virus infection. Usually it is an acute self limiting infection. In approximately 5 to 15 percent of cases it fails to resolve and the affected individual then become persistent carriers of the virus" (Park, 1997, p. 158).

"In one study case fatality rate of hepatitis B was 15.6 percent" (Park, 1997, p. 159).

In lobar pneumonia, if patients are not treated by antibiotic, then

> The fever persists at 104°–105°F for an average of 7–8 days (and on rare occasions for 11–12 days). The patient continues to be extremely ill with a hot dry skin, a painful cough, considerable sleeplessness and exhaustion and takes little nourishment. About the seventh or eighth day the fever as also the pulse and respiration rate, in favourable cases, terminates by crisis, falling to normal in the course of a few hours. This is accompanied by marked general improvement, the pulse respiration ratio returns to normal. (Warner, 1964, pp. 195–196)

Conclusively, we can say that in tropical diseases the maximum number of patients recovers spontaneously without effective treatment but may take longer duration. A small percentage of patients may die from tropical diseases without treatment. We can get a 100% cure rate if diseases are treated properly. In nontropical diseases like hypertension, diabetes, cancer, asthma, etc., if diseases are not treated properly, then there is gradual deterioration and death but this may take years. In nontropical diseases like myocardial infarction, cardiac failure, cerebral stroke, kidney failure, patients die sooner or later in the absence of treatment. In chronic diseases, there is a possibility of fluctuations in severity. Remissions and exacerbations are also there. Without clinically controlled trials, these fluctuations give the wrong impression of cure.

A percentage of the population reacts positively to placebo.

> Placebo medicine is a vehicle for cure by suggestion and surprisingly often successful, if only temporarily. All treatments carry placebo effects ... A placebo reactor is an individual who reports change of physical or mental state after taking a pharmacologically

Chapter fifty five: Hahnemann accepted failure 229

> inert substance. Placebo reactors are suggestible
> people are likely to respond favourably to any treat-
> ment. They have misled doctors into making false
> therapeutic claims. Negative reactors, who develop
> adverse effects when given a placebo ... Some 35%
> of the physically ill and 40% of mentally ill respond
> to placebo. (Bennett & Brown, 2003, p. 23)

Nontropical diseases like cardiac problems, diabetes, renal diseases, carcinomas, strokes usually begin in elderly people. Children, adolescents, and young persons usually do not suffer from these diseases. They suffer mainly from tropical diseases which usually resolve spontaneously in a large number of patients.

Hahnemann put all nonsexually transmitted diseases in one group and said they are due to psora. He prescribed different antipsoric homeopathic drugs for different diseases according to the homeopathic principle. He said,

> The eruption is only to be removed by internal heal-
> ing and curative remedies which change the state
> of the whole, then also the eruption which is based
> on the internal disease will be cured and healed of
> itself without the help of any external remedy and
> frequently more quickly than it could be done by
> external remedies. (Hahnemann, 1999, p. 174)

He also said,

> The great truth is established that all chronic ail-
> ments, all great and the greatest, long continuing
> disease (excepting the few venereal ones) spring
> from psora alone and only find their thorough cure
> in the cure of psora; they are consequently to be
> healed mostly only by antipsoric remedies i.e., by
> those remedies which in their provings as to their
> pure action on the healthy human body manifest
> most of the symptoms which are most frequently
> perceived in latent as well as in developed psora.
> (Hahnemann, 1999, p. 203)

Hahnemann thought all diseases are due to psora, syphilis, and psychoses. He wrongly accepted that he was able to cure diseases by homeopathic method. The fact was not obvious to Hahnemann. He did not have knowledge about pathology, etiology, diagnosis, and treatment of disease. He also did not know, "Clinical evaluation, pharmacokinetic, and pharmacodynamic study of a drug and how a drug is discovered".

More than 60% of patients from tropical diseases are cured spontaneously without any effective treatment. It is certain that without effective treatment some patients may die and in remaining patients, morbidity, severity, and duration of disease will be greater. With the help of modern medical effective treatment, morbidity, severity, and duration of disease are decreased with cent percent cure. Spontaneous recovery in a large percentage of the population gave the wrong message to the world that homeopathy is effective. Similar unnecessary reputation is also being earned on similar grounds by many useless therapies.

Placebo reaction also gives a transitory curative effect which helps in the establishment of a reputation of unnecessary and useless pathies. To understand this fact that homeopathy is ineffective, knowledge of medical science is must. If a person is glorifying any pathy after seeing a curative effect in one or two patients, it means he does not know anything regarding medical science. That's why I say Hahnemann was wrong. Homeopathy was wrong. It works as a placebo only. Homeopathy has no therapeutic utility.

Hahnemann also accepted failure. He said that he was not able to cure all chronic patients. He also said, "Homeopathy is ineffective in certain conditions." What are those factors, which make homeopathy ineffective according to Hahnemann? Hahnemann said,

> These same events if they occur to a person already a chronic patient may not only augment his disease and increase the difficulty of curing it but if they break in on him violently may make his disease incurable, if the untoward circumstances are not suddenly changed for the better. (Hahnemann, 1999, p. 193)

He writes about factors that are responsible for failure of homeopathic treatment. "An innocent man can with less injury to his life pass ten years in bodily torments in the bastille or on the galleys rather than pass some months in all bodily comfort in an unhappy marriage or with a remorseful conscience"(Hahnemann, 1999, p. 193).

Regarding factors that increase duration of disease and decrease effectiveness of homeopathic treatment, Hahnemann writes, "Excessive hardships, laboring in swamps, great bodily injury and wounds, excess of

Chapter fifty five: Hahnemann accepted failure   231

cold and heat and even the unsatisfied hunger of poverty and its unwholesome foods" (Hahnemann, 1999, p. 193).

According to Hahnemann, contempt and poverty are also responsible for producing ailments. He tells,

> A psora slumbering within which still allows the favourite of a prince to live with the appearance of almost blooming health unfolds quickly into a chronic ailment of the body or distracts his mental organs into insanity, when by a change of fortune he is hurled from his brilliant pinnacle and is exposed to contempt and poverty. (Hahnemann, 1999, pp. 193–194)

Hahnemann also said, "The sudden death of a son causes the tender mother, already in ill health, an incurable suppuration of the lungs or a cancer of the breast" (Hahnemann, 1999, p. 194).

Hahnemann accepted failure in the treatment in the following words, "How difficult it is and how seldom will the best anti-psoric treatment do anything to relieve such unfortunates" (Hahnemann, 1999, p. 194). He says that all imaginable chronic sufferings can develop from uninterrupted grief and vexation.

> If grief and vexation continually beat in upon him and it is out of the power of the physician to effect a lasting removal of these most active destroyers of life, he had better give up the treatment and leave the patient to his fate for even the most masterly management of the case with the remedies that are the most exquisite and the best adopted to the bodily ailment will avail nothing, nothing at all, with a chronic patient thus exposed to continue sorrow and vexation. (Hahnemann, 1999, p. 195)

Hahnemann agreed that grief and vexation prevent the curative effect of homeopathic drugs. It has even been said by Hahnemann, "It is better to leave the patient to his fate rather than to treat when the patient is in grief and vexation". Vexation means a state of being annoyed and worried. When a person is in severe chronic ailments, he would be definitely in grief and vexation. Hahnemann says this patient cannot be cured. According to him, first grief and vexation should be removed, and then disease will be cured. But this is not the fact. Fact is that disease should be removed first then grief and vexation will subside automatically.

232   *Homeopathy*

Hahnemann rationalized failure of treatment. He produced unnecessary pretense. When diseases have been cured spontaneously, he gave credit to homeopathy. When diseases have not been cured, he pointed out those factors that were not actually responsible for failure. For example, in one example, he said, suppuration of lung and cancer of breast are incurable due to sudden death of a patient's son. Today a person having knowledge of diseases knows very well that death of a son cannot be made responsible for incurable suppuration of lung and carcinoma of breast. In this way, we can say, Hahnemann accepted failure but produced wrong arguments. Conclusively, we can say that grief and vexation cannot make disease incurable, if successful treatment is available. Hahnemann says such things that indicate only failure of homeopathic treatment.

Other causes of incurability of chronic diseases are as mentioned by Hahnemann.

> Almost as near, and often nearer yet, to incurability are the chronic diseases especially with great and rich men, who for some years besides the use of mineral bath, have passed through the hands of various, often of many, allopathic physicians…. And after the continuation of such irrational medical assaults on the organism for several years it becomes almost quite incurable. (Hahnemann, 1999, pp. 195–196)

I agree that old allopathic treatment was injurious to health and blood of the patient was made to flow by bleeding, leeches, etc. or medicine was prescribed to evacuate the contents of stomach and intestine. These procedures destroyed life acutely but after the gap of a considerable time things changed. Toxic and harmful effects of old allopathic treatment should have disappeared after some time. If homeopathic treatment was effective, then it could have cured these patients. They should have been managed by homeopathic treatment. But Hahnemann was not able to manage these patients and he illogically projected mineral bath and allopathic treatment as causes of failure.

Other causes of failure of homeopathic treatment are ridiculous. Hahnemann writes,

> Great hindrance to a cure of far advanced chronic diseases is often found in the debility and weakness into which youth fall who are spoiled by rich parents, being carried away by their superabundance and wantonness and seduced by wicked companions through destructive passions and excesses through revealing abuse of the sexual

Chapter fifty five: Hahnemann accepted failure

> instinct, gambling etc. without the least regard for
> life and for conscience bodies originally robust are
> debilitate by such vices into mere semblances of
> humanity. (Hahnemann, 1999, p. 200)

This para says that if a patient is a gambler or spoiled youth of rich parents, it cannot be managed by homeopathic treatment.

Hahnemann also mentioned a typical cause of failure. This cause is not related to the patient but this cause is related to disease. He tells,

> There is nevertheless found at times, especially with
> the lower classes of patients a peculiar obstruction
> to the cure, which lies in the source of the malady
> itself where the psora after repeated infections
> and a repeated external repression of the resulting
> eruptions had developed gradually from its inter-
> nal state into one of more severe chronic ailments
> (Hahnemann, 1999, p. 201).

He also writes, "If patients are aged or debilitated, chances of improvement are very less" (Hahnemann, 1999, p. 201). Here Hahnemann writes very clearly, if disease is chronic and severe, then chances of improvement are very rare. If patients are aged or debilitated, then chances of cure are less. It shows Hahnemann himself admits that chances of failure of homeopathic treatment are very high.

Prescription of new drugs or repetition of the same medicine also interferes with recovery. As Hahnemann says,

> Once a medicine, because it was selected in a cor-
> rect homeopathic manner, is acting well of usefully,
> which is seen by the 8th or 10th day, then an hour or
> even half a day may come when a moderate homeo-
> pathic aggravation again takes place ... The dose
> will then probably have exhausted its favourable
> action about the fortieth or fiftieth day and before
> that time it would be injudicious and an obstruction
> to the progress of the cure to give any other medi-
> cine. (Hahnemann, 1999, p. 209)

> The whole treatment will amount to nothing.
> Another antipsoric remedy which may be ever so
> useful, but is prescribed too early and before the
> cessation of the action of the present remedy or a
> new dose of the same remedy which is still usefully

234   *Homeopathy*

> acting can in no case replace the good effect which
> has been lost through the interruption of the com-
> plete action of the preceding remedy which was
> acting usefully which can hardly be again replaced.
> (Hahnemann, 1999, p. 213)

In some cases, "Every new medicine and also a new dose of the same medicine would interrupt the work of improvement and cause new ailments, an interference which often cannot be repaired for a long time" (Hahnemann, 1999, p. 215).

If a homeopath gives new antipsoric medicine or repeats the same medicine within 30 or 40 days of first dose in treatment of chronic diseases, it will be the definite cause of failure of treatment, Hahnemann says. He says repetition of dose of the same medicine or new drug in chronic diseases will interfere in recovery or create new diseases, if used within 30 or 40 days. Followers of homeopathy are using frequent doses. They are against Hahnemann. Are they treating patients or are they creating new ailments?

Hahnemann also provided a list of conditions which disturb the treatment. He enumerated overloading the stomach, disorder of the stomach from fat, nausea, and inclination to vomit, disorder of the stomach with gastric fever, chilliness and cold, fright and timidity, vexation, sadness caused by the fright, vexation which causes anger, heat irritation, indignation with silent internal mortification, unsuccessful love with quite grief, unhappy love with jealousy, a severe cold a cold which is followed by suffocative fits, cold followed by pains and inclination to weep, cold with consequent coryza, contusions, and wounds inflicted by blunt instruments, burning of the skin, weakness from loss of fluids and blood, homesickness with redness of the cheeks (Hahnemann, 1999, pp. 224–225).

Hahnemann also says that large or strong doses of a drug also create hurdles in treatment. He says,

> A medicine even though it may be homeopathically
> suited to the case of disease, does harm in every
> dose that is too large and in strong doses it does
> more harm, the greater its homeopathically and
> higher the potency selected, and it does much more
> injury than any equally large does of a medicine
> that is unhomeopathic and in no respect adapted to
> morbid state (allopathic). Too large doses of an accu-
> rately chosen homeopathic medicine and especially
> when frequently repeated bring about much trouble
> as a rule. (Hahnemann, 1921/2017, p. 228)

Chapter fifty five: Hahnemann accepted failure   235

Hahnemann also advised many precautions which should be taken during homeopathic treatment otherwise treatment will not be effective. "Obstacles to cure is so much more necessary in the case of patients affected by chronic diseases, as their diseases are usually aggravated by such noxious influences and other diseases, causing errors in the diet and regimen which often pass unnoticed" (Hahnemann, 1921/2017, p. 214).

> These are coffee, fine Chinese and other herb teas, beer … all kind of punch, spiced chocolate, odorous waters and perfumes of many kinds, strong scented flowers in the apartment, tooth powders, and essences and perfumed sachets, compounded of drug, highly spiced dishes and sauces, spiced cakes and ices … all vegetables possessing medicinal properties, celery, onions, old cheese … heated rooms, woollen clothing next the skin, a sedentary life in close apartments or the frequent indulgence in mere passive exercise (such as riding, driving or swinging), prolonged suckling, taking a long siesta in a recumbent posture in bed, sitting up long at night uncleanliness, unnatural debauchery, enervation by reading obscene books, reading while lying down, onanism or imperfect or suppressed intercourse in order to prevent conception, subjects of anger, grief or vexation, a passion for play, over-exertion of mind or body especially after meals, dwelling in marshy districts, damp-rooms, penurious living etc. All these things must be as far as possible avoided or removed, in order that the cure may not be obstructed or rendered impossible. (Hahnemann, 1921/2017, pp. 214–215)

Hahnemann also mentioned astronomical influence. He writes,

> During the treatment of chronic diseases by antipsoric remedies we often need the other non-antipsoric store of medicines in cases where epidemic diseases or intermediate arising usually from meteoric and telluric causes attack our chronic patients so not only temporarily disturb the treatment but even interrupt it for longer time. (Hahnemann, 1999, p. 235)

Hahnemann mentioned many factors for failure of homeopathic treatment. It is not correct. Reality is different from what has been said by Hahnemann. Actually, now I am explaining. The diseases which resolved spontaneously, Hahnemann gave credit to homeopathy. Diseases that were not resolved spontaneously were attributed to many other factors. He observed in patients that gambling, onions, perfumes, flowers, tooth powders, vegetables, meteoric body, rest and sleep taken in the early afternoon, grief and vexation, etc., interfered in homeopathic treatment. A person having knowledge of science and diseases knows very well that these factors mentioned by Hahnemann do not influence recovery of diseases. In fact, Hahnemann was wrong. Homeopathy has only a placebo effect.

Homeopathy got good results only in those patients who were being deteriorated by old allopathic methods especially in acute pyrexial and in acute diarrheal diseases. In these cases, actually homeopathy was not effective but old allopathic methods had to be stopped which were dangerous and fatal to patients suffering from acute feverish and acute diarrheal diseases. In management of smallpox, "fluid deficit should be replaced by administration of appropriate solutions" (Ray, 1983, p. 1120).

In the treatment of typhoid, "Nursing care and attention to nutritional requirements are important. Laxatives and enemas should be avoided" (Guerrant & Hook, 1983, p. 961). In dysentery, a fluid or semi-fluid low roughage diet should be given depending on the severity of diarrhea but if this is severe, it will be necessary to replace the water and electrolyte loss by intravenous therapy (Griffin et al., 1999, p. 127). In whooping cough, "When the illness is of long duration and vomiting is frequent, skilled nursing will be required to maintain nutrition, especially in infants and young children" (Griffin et al., 1999, p. 123).

When persons suffer from fever and diarrhea, adequate nutrition and water, and electrolyte balance are very necessary to prevent morbidity and mortality. If dehydration is produced in these patients by vomiting and purgation and blood is removed from the body, then these procedures become highly dangerous and detrimental to the body and increase morbidity and mortality, as advised by old allopathy. Then chances of spontaneous recovery are over. In measles, cholera, scarlet fever, whooping cough, dysentery, and typhoid, chances of spontaneous recovery are great. When in these patients dehydration is produced or blood is removed as advised by the old allopathic method of treatment, chances of complications and death are very much increased. Homeopathic methods did not provide cure in these patients but protected the patients from the damaging effect of old allopathy, prevalent at that time. That's why homeopathy got a reputation as a curing agent. Homeopathy itself has no therapeutic ability but replaced old allopathy that's why homeopathy prevented the exhausting debilitating effect of old allopathy and got a false reputation as a curative and highly effective therapeutic method.

Chapter fifty five: Hahnemann accepted failure   237

Nowadays the concept of old allopathy has totally changed. Today, developed medical science is based on scientific studies, experiments, and controlled observations. Purgation, blood removal, and concept of plethora are not accepted today. Electrolytes and fluid are administered in dehydrated conditions and blood is also administered when required. Knowledge of different branches of science is being used today in the medical field. New advanced methods of investigation are being utilized today. Morbidity and mortality are also reducing day by day. Today we have vast knowledge. Acceptance of homeopathy indicates our ignorance, lack of knowledge, unscientific approach, and inability to understand science. Prevalence of homeopathy in 2022 A.D. is against society, against humanity, against knowledge, and against intelligence. Societies and nations are losing money, time, and lives by supporting homeopathy.

References

Bennett, P. N., & Brown, M. J. (2003). *Clinical pharmacology* (9th ed.). Delhi, India: E.L.B.S & Churchill Livingstone.

Griffin, G. E., Sissons, J. G. P., Chiodini, P. L., & Mitchell, D. M. (1999). Diseases due to infection. In C. Haslett, E. R. Chillers, J. A. A. Hunter, & N. A. Boon (Eds.), *Davidson's principles and practice of medicine* (18th ed., pp. 56–190). Edinburgh, United Kingdom: Churchill Livingstone.

Guerrant, R. L., & Hook, E. (1983). Salmonella infection. In R. G. Petersdorf, R. D. Adams, E. Braunwald, K. J. Isselbacher, J. B. Martin, & J. D. Wilson (Eds.), *Harrison's principle of internal medicine* (10th ed., pp. 957–965). New Delhi, India: McGraw Hill.

Hahnemann, S. (1999). *The chronic diseases (theoretical part)* (Reprint ed.). New Delhi, India: B Jain Publishers.

Hahnemann, S. (2017). *Organon of medicine* (6th ed.) (W. Boericke, Trans.). New Delhi, India: B. Jain Publishers. (Original work published in 1921).

Park, K. (1997). *Park's textbook of preventive and social medicine* (15th ed.). Jabalpur, India: Banarsidas Bhanot Publisher.

Ray, C. G. (1983). Smallpox, vaccinia and cowpox. In R. G. Petersdorf, R. D. Adams, E. Braunwald, K. J. Isselbacher, J. B. Martin, & J. D. Wilson (Eds.), *Harrison's principle of internal medicine* (10th ed., pp. 1118–1121). New Delhi, India: McGraw Hill.

Warner, E. C. (Ed.) (1964). *Savill's system of clinical medicine* (14th ed.). London, United Kingdom: Edward Arnold Publisher.

chapter fifty six

Research on homeopathy

Basic concept of this book: homeopathy – an illusion of effectiveness: fifty six

Hahnemann basic principles have been analyzed on the basis of knowledge of basic medical science in previous chapters. They all are inaccurate, wrong, and unscientific. When principles of homeopathy are wrong, then a drug produced on the basis of these principles cannot be effective. It means all homeopathic drugs are useless and ineffective. They cannot cure any disease. Clinical trials also prove that homeopathic drugs are not therapeutically effective.

Explanation

Hahnemann's basic principles have been analyzed on the basis of knowledge of basic medical science in previous chapters. They all are inaccurate, wrong, and unscientific. German physician Samuel Hahnemann framed wrong principles due to unavailability of knowledge in 1796. Basic medical science opposes all principles of homeopathy.

When principles of homeopathy are wrong, then a drug produced on the basis of these principles cannot be effective. It means all homeopathic drugs are useless and ineffective. They cannot cure any disease. Clinical trials also prove that homeopathic drugs are not therapeutically effective. Clinical trials and research studies also confirm this absolute truth. Conclusions of many researches and lclinical trials are being mentioned here to see effectiveness of homeopathy.

1. **Smith (2012)** – Smith writes in his research paper regarding dilution of homeopathic remedies,

> To receive just one molecule of the diluted agent from a fairly standard homeopathic in dilution of 1×10^{30}, the patient would have to consume over 30,000 litres of the homeopathic solution. And many homeopathic medicines are diluted to even greater extremes, ranging up to 1×10^{400}, meaning that to receive just one molecule of agent the patient would

DOI: 10.1201/9781003228622-56

have to consume more matter than is present within the universe.

Smith also said,

It is unethical to advise for homeopathic treatment. The modest duty on individual citizens to reject homeopathy only applies where those concerned possess reliable knowledge about homeopathy. In this respect, it is the prescribers and (true) proponents of homeopathy who carry the lion's share of ethical responsibility. By prescribing ineffective medicine and promulgating falsehoods about homeopathic efficacy, it is these advocates, as opposed to the users of homeopathy, who are guilty of serious unethical behavior.

Smith also described, "Homeopathy cannot work and does not work, I suggest that my utilitarian analysis of homeopathy remains valid. Homeopathy is ethically unacceptable and ought to be actively rejected by health-care professionals".

2. **Shang et al. (2005)** – Shang et al. selected 110 placebo-controlled trials of homeopathy and 110 trials in conventional medicine matched to homeopathy trials were randomly selected from the Cochrane Controlled Trials Register. Bias effects were examined.

Biases are present in placebo-controlled trials of both homoeopathy and conventional medicine. When account was taken for these biases in the analysis, there was weak evidence for a specific effect of homoeopathic remedies, but strong evidence for specific effects of conventional interventions. This finding is compatible with the notion that the clinical effects of homoeopathy are placebo effects.

3. **Ernst (2002)** – In this research paper, Ernst is attempting to clarify the effectiveness of homeopathy based on recent systematic reviews. In this publication, 17 articles fulfilled the inclusion/exclusion criteria. Six of them are related to reanalyses of meta-analysis. Eleven independent systematic reviews were located. Collectively they failed to provide strong evidence in favor of homeopathy. There was

Chapter fifty six: Research on homeopathy 241

no condition which responds convincingly better to homeopathic treatment than to placebo or other control interventions. Similarly, there was no homeopathic remedy that was demonstrated to yield clinical effects that are convincingly different from placebo. This research paper concluded,

> The hypothesis that any given homeopathic remedy leads to clinical effects that are relevantly different from placebo or superior to other control interventions for any medical condition, is not supported by evidence from systematic reviews. Until more compelling results are available, homeopathy cannot be viewed as an evidence-based form of therapy.

According to this paper, homeopathy cannot be recommended for use in clinical practice.

4. **Aabel (2000)** – The objective of this research paper was to determine efficacy of homeopathic medicine, Betula 30c at reducing symptoms of pollen allergy in patients sensitive to birch pollen. It was a double-blind, randomized, placebo-controlled trial done by Aable. He concluded,

> Surprisingly, the verum treated patients fared worse than the placebo group; they used more rescue medication and had higher symptom scores during these three days. Homeopaths might attribute the findings to a putative aggravation response, but the results certainly do not lend support to the usefulness of the tested prophylactic approach, under conditions of low allergen exposure.

5. **Baum and Ernst (2009)** – Baum and Ernst rightly expressed their view in their paper that these homeopathy supporters are not supporters of knowledge and science. They said, "These individuals have a conflict of interest more powerful than the requirement for scientific integrity". Michael Baum writes in his research paper that homeopathy is among the worst examples of faith-based medicine that gathers shrill support of celebrities and other powerful lobbies in place of a genuine and humble wish to explore the limits of our knowledge using the scientific method. Authors coordinate principles of homeopathy and science and conclusively said, "If homeopathy is correct, much of physics, chemistry, and pharmacology must be incorrect".

Authors also said about those trials that showed effectiveness of homeopathic remedies,

> Homeopathy cannot work and that positive evidence reflects publication bias or design flaw until proved otherwise. So far homeopathy has failed to demonstrate efficacy in randomized controlled trials and systematic reviews of well designed studies. Homeopathic physicians seem to clutch on to the straws of a series of poorly designed or underpowered studies to retain their credibility or claim.

6. **Davey(2015) – National Health and Medical Research Council (NHMRC) Australia** – NHMRC Australia (2015) for the first time thoroughly reviewed 225 research papers, 57 systematic reviews, and a high-quality type of study that synthesizes it to make a number of strong, overall findings on homeopathy.

   This review used standardized, accepted methods for assessing the quality and reliability of evidence for whether or not a therapy is effective for treating health conditions and concluded, "That there are no health conditions for which there is reliable evidence that homeopathy is effective. People who choose homeopathy may put their health at risk if they reject or delay treatments for which there is good evidence for safety and effectiveness". This report also analyzed studies and reported that homeopathy was effective and concluded that the quality of those studies was poor and suffered serious flaws in their design and did not have enough participants to support the idea that homeopathy worked any better than a sugar pill, the report found.

7. **Ramesh (2020)** – It is an article by Ramesh, in response to the use of homeopathy to prevent infection. As the title of this article says, "Forget coronavirus, homoeopathy can't cure anything. It's a placebo, at best". He explained,

> Most health experts, from the World Health Organisation (WHO), to the US Department of Health and Human Services and Britain's National Health Service cite research and express scepticism. They discourage its use as an alternative to conventional medicine for life-threatening diseases, and see it as a harmless placebo at best and a purveyor of potentially lethal concoctions at worst. Several countries like Britain and France do not allow

Chapter fifty six: Research on homeopathy

government funding in the field, while Australia conducted a thorough review and declared it pseudoscience. Spain has proposed banning it for being dangerous.

In this article, it has been also said that research work has shown that homeopathy is ineffective in treating illness and studies show positive findings were not conducted properly or used insufficient evidence. Author also explained, "National medical and health bodies in Russia, Australia, and Europe have warned against homoeopathy. Many countries have conducted comprehensive research and have ultimately decided that it doesn't work".

8. **Cucherat et al. (2000)** – In this research paper, M. Cucherat et al. used systemic review and meta-analysis, to see the efficacy of homeopathic treatment in patients with any disease. One hundred and eighteen randomized trials were identified and evaluated for inclusion. They said,

> There is some evidence that homeopathic treatments are more effective than placebo; however, the strength of this evidence is low because of the low methodological quality of the trials. Studies of high methodological quality were more likely to be negative than the lower quality studies. Further high quality studies are needed to confirm these results.

In this study, it has been also concluded, "Low methodological quality of research may give results in favor of homeopathy. But such a result cannot be accepted in scientific studies".

9. **UK Science and Technology Committee (2010)** – House of Commons, Science and Technology Committee (UK), Fourth Report on Homeopathy, regarding the policy on National Health Service (NHS) funding and provision of homeopathy (2010) clearly says, (1) Homeopathy should be stopped and Government should not invest money on homeopathy treatment and further research on homeopathy is not required. (2) We consider that conclusions about the evidence on the efficacy of homeopathy should be derived from well-designed and rigorous randomized controlled trials (RCTs) (Paragraph 20). (3) We expect the conclusions on the evidence for the efficacy of homeopathy to give particular weight to properly conducted meta-analyses and systematic reviews of RCTs (Paragraph 25). (4) The systematic reviews and meta-analyses conclusively demonstrated that homeopathic products performed no

better than placebos (Paragraph 70). (5) There has been enough testing of homeopathy and plenty of evidence showing that it is not efficacious. Competition for research funding is fierce and we cannot see how further research on the efficacy of homeopathy is justified in the face of competing priorities (Paragraph 77). (6) We recommend that if personal health budgets proceed beyond the pilot stage the government should not allow patients to buy nonevidence-based treatments such as homeopathy with public money (Paragraph 104). (7) When the NHS funds homeopathy, it endorses it. The government should stop allowing the funding of homeopathy on the NHS (Paragraph 110).

10. **Mathie et al. (2014)** – Sometimes small trials of individualized homeopathic treatment showed greater than placebo effect. But any decisive conclusion cannot be drawn due to poor quality of evidence and small sample size. This is the story of all clinical trials which show positive effects of homeopathic remedies.

In this study, 32 eligible RCTs, studied 24 different medical conditions in total and focused systematic review and meta-analysis of RCTs of individualized homeopathic treatment, were done. They tested the hypothesis that the result of an individualized homeopathic treatment using homeopathic medicines is different from that of placebo. Authors explained,

> Medicines prescribed in individualised homeopathy may have small, specific treatment effects. Findings are consistent with sub-group data available in a previous global systematic review. The low or unclear overall quality of the evidence prompts caution in interpreting the findings. New high-quality RCT research is necessary to enable more decisive interpretation.

11. **Linde et al. (1997)** – The aim of this trial is to assess whether the clinical effect reported in RCT of homeopathic remedies is equivalent to that reported for placebo. Double-blind and/or randomized, placebo-controlled trials of clinical conditions were considered. A review of 185 trials identified 119 that met the inclusion criteria. Eighty-nine had adequate data for meta-analysis. They said,

> The results of our meta-analysis are not compatible with the hypothesis that the clinical effects of homeopathy are completely due to placebo.

Chapter fifty six: Research on homeopathy 245

However, we found insufficient evidence from these studies that homeopathy is clearly efficacious for any single clinical condition. Further research on homeopathy is warranted provided it is rigorous and systematic.

12. **Shaddel et al. (2014)** – In this research paper, the role of homeopathy to treat psychiatric disorders has been studied. Twelve relevant clinical trials were identified and included in this study.

This paper says, "The currently available evidence is neither conclusive nor comprehensive enough to give us a clear picture for the use of homeopathy in patients with intellectual disabilities. There are large gaps in the body of evidence concerning the role of homeopathy in the treatment of common disorders in intellectual disability, such as autism, challenging behavior or developmental arrest in childhood".

13. **Kleijnen et al. (1991)** – In this work, the aim of researchers was to establish whether there was evidence of the efficacy of homeopathy from meta-analysis of controlled trials in humans. They assessed the methodological quality of 107 controlled trials in 96 published reports. In this study,

The evidence of clinical trials was positive but not sufficient to draw definitive conclusions because most trials were of low methodological quality and because of the unknown role of publication bias. This indicates that there was a legitimate case for further evaluation of homoeopathy, but only by means of well performed trials.

14. **Subhranil and Munmun (2013)** – The aim of this review was to summarize treatment effects of individualized homeopathy in headaches and migraine. Randomized controlled trials comparing individualized homeopathic treatment strategy with placebo were eligible. Trials providing sufficient data were analyzed in a quantitative meta-analysis. A total of four randomized placebo-controlled trials involving 390 patients were considered for the analysis. "There was no statistically significant difference in favor of homeopathy. The results of our meta-analysis are not compatible with the notion that homeopathy has significant effects beyond placebo".

15. **European Academies' Science Advisory Council (EASAC, 2017)** – The academics and scientists of the EU member states joined together

246 *Homeopathy*

to establish EASAC in 2001. EASAC is a group of independent Europe's leading scientists to guide EU policy for the benefit of society. It brings together the National Academies of Science of the EU Member States, Norway, Switzerland, and UK, including 29 national and international scientific academies, including the Royal Society (UK) and Royal Swedish Academy of Sciences. Through EASAC, the academies and scientists work together to provide independent, expert, evidence-based advice to European institutions. EASAC is publishing this statement regarding the use of homeopathic products on Wed, 20 September 2017. EASAC makes the following statement on homeopathy,

> A new evaluation from EASAC confirms, there is no robust, reproducible evidence that homeopathic products are effective for any known diseases, even if there is sometimes a placebo effect. Moreover, homeopathy can actually be harmful: by delaying or deterring a patient from seeking appropriate, evidence-based, medical attention and by undermining patient and public confidence in scientific evidence.

EASAC also explained,

> From analysis of the appropriately controlled, verifiable evidence base, any claimed efficacy of homeopathic products in clinical use can be explained by the placebo effect or attributed to poor study design, random variation, regression towards the mean, or publication bias. While the placebo effect can be of value to the patient. The scientific claims made for homeopathy are implausible and inconsistent with established concepts from chemistry and physics.

16. **Güell (2018)** – Spain has planned to ban pseudo-therapies from universities and health centers.

> Government has put forward a plan to fight the rise of pseudo-therapies such as homeopathy, which promise to have a positive health impact but have no scientific evidence to support their claims. The proposal,

Chapter fifty six: Research on homeopathy   247

unprecedented in the European Union, aims to eliminate so-called alternative therapies from health centers and universities. The plan comes two months
after 400 Spanish scientists signed an open letter call-
ing for action against pseudo-science.

The government also said that besides not working, pseudo-
therapies like homeopathy negatively affect health by perpetuat-
ing illnesses, causing others, or even increasing the risk of death.
According to the government, they do this by encouraging a person
to substitute or delay taking conventional medicine of proven safety
and effectiveness. "Public and private establishments that include
pseudo-therapies will not be able to call themselves health centers",
explained the Health Minister. Their presence in these spaces gives
the idea that they have a therapeutic use. The first thing we have to
make clear is that they do not. And if they do not, it makes no sense
for them to be there, officials said.

Government is also planning to make legislation to stop public-
ity that promotes alternative therapy services, products, events, or
anything else relating to pseudo-therapies and to remove any degree
that includes pseudo-therapies from the country's universities.

17. **Dearden (2017) and Litvinova (2017)** – Lizzie Dearden mentioned
in the *Independent* newspaper that the Russian Academy of Sciences
in Russia has also declared that homeopathy has no scientific basis
and endangers people who use it.

A memorandum issued by the Commission
Against Pseudoscience and falsification of Scientific
Research described the 'treatments' as pseudosci-
entific, saying that attempts to verify their success had failed for over 200 years. Homeopathy
is not innocuous. Patients spend heavily on non-
performing drugs and neglected means of treatment with proven effectiveness. This can lead to
adverse outcomes, including death of the patient.
(Dearden, 2017)

Scientists from the Russian Academy of Sciences
(RAS) warn that the fad poses dangers. Patients who
reject standard medicine in favor of unproven
homeopathic cures put their lives at risk, they wrote
in their latest memorandum. The principles of
homeopathy contradict known chemical, physical

and biological laws, while there are no persuasive scientific trials proving its effectiveness, the RAS commission on pseudoscience said in a document released in December. (Litvinova, 2017)

18. **Agence France-Presse in Paris (2019) – A report published in** *The Guardian* **says,**

> In France, the French government has announced it will stop reimbursing patients for homeopathic treatment from 2021 after a major national study concluded the alternative medicine had no proven benefit. The health minister, Agnès Buzyn, a former doctor who has vowed to place scientific rigour at the heart of policy, said she had made the decision after a damning verdict on homeopathy by the national health authority in June.

This report also describes, "France's National Authority for Health (HAS) concluded at the end of June that there was no benefit to the medicine, saying it had not scientifically demonstrated sufficient effectiveness to justify a reimbursement". Report also says, "In Britain, the National Health Service also decided in 2017 to stop funding homeopathic care. Public health systems in other EU countries such as Sweden and Austria do not support the treatment".

19. **The National Association of Statutory Health Insurance Physicians (NASHIP, 2019). DW News –** In Germany also, doctors are against the funding of homeopathy due to ineffectiveness.

> The head of the main doctors' association and the SPD's health specialist have called for an end to refunds for homeopathy treatments in Germany. Their calls follow a similar move in France. The head of the National Association of Statutory Health Insurance Physicians (KBV), which represents 150,000 doctors and psychotherapists in Germany, said that health insurance companies should not fund homeopathic services. There is insufficient scientific evidence for the efficacy of homeopathic procedures.

20. **Belluz (2016) –** According to this report, "The US government is also finally telling people and consumers that homeopathy is not

Chapter fifty six: Research on homeopathy   249

effective, it is a sham only. Companies that make homeopathic products will be required to spell out that their products are not based on scientific evidence. Clinical trials have established homeopathy is not effective."

This report also says, "The United States government only recently decided to clamp down on these bogus treatments, with a new policy from the Federal Trade Commission. The FTC's policy statement explains that the agency will now ask that the makers of homeopathic drugs present reliable scientific evidence for their health claims if they want to sell them to consumers on the US market".

21. **Zonas et al. (2001)** – In this research paper, the author did systematic review, comparing the quality of clinical-trial research in homeopathy to a sample of research on conventional therapies. All clinical trials on homeopathic treatments, published between 1945 and 1995 in English, were selected. All clinical trials were evaluated. Fifty-nine studies met the inclusion criteria. The authors concluded,

> That there was practically no replication of or overlap in the conditions studied and most studies were relatively small and done at a single-site. Compared to research on conventional therapies the overall quality of studies in homeopathy was worse and only slightly improved in more recent years.
>
> Clinical homeopathic research is clearly in its infancy with most studies using poor sampling and measurement techniques, few subjects, single sites and no replication.

22. **Vithoulkas (2017)** – In this article, Vithoulkas discussed the serious mistakes in meta-analysis of homeopathic research. The main focus was related to the use of basic homeopathic principles in clinical trials and effectiveness of homeopathic treatment.

> The examination of most of the homeopathic trials showed that studies rarely account for homeopathic principles, in order to assess the effectiveness of the treatment. The main flaw was that trials reflect the point of view that the treatment with a specific remedy could be administered in a particular disease. However, homeopathy aims to treat the whole person, rather than the diseases and each case has to

be treated individually or with an individualized remedy. Furthermore, the commonly known events during the course of homeopathic treatment, such as initial aggravation 'and a symptom-shift' were not considered in almost all the studies. Thus, only a few trials were eligible for meta-analyses, if at all.

According to principles of homeopathy, prescription of new drugs or repetition of the same medicine also interferes in the recovery from diseases. Hahnemann says that a homeopathic medicine may take 10–50 days to show its full effect and before that time it would be injudicious and an obstruction to the progress of the cure to repeat the same medicine or give any other medicine. Author rightly criticized the methods of homeopathic trials.

Author also said, "In severe chronic conditions, the homeopath may need to correctly prescribe a series of remedies before the improvement is apparent. Such a second or third prescription should take place only after evaluating the effects of the previous remedies. Again, this rule has also been ignored in most studies".

23. **Editorial, *Lancet* (2005)** – In the editorial of *Lancet* in 2005, after publication of Aijing Shang and colleagues systematic evaluation of 110 placebo-controlled trials of homeopathy and 110 trials in conventional medicine matched to homeopathy trials, it has been written, "it is the end of homeopathy. In this systematic evaluation homeopathy was no better than placebo". Editor writes, "This unnecessary debate on homeopathy continues, despite 150 years of unfavourable findings".

Editor also mentioned one psychological fact, "We see things not as they are, but as we are. This observation is also true for health-care consumers, who may see homeopathy as a holistic alternative to a disease-focused, technology-driven medical model. It is the attitudes of patients and providers that engender alternative-therapy-seeking behaviors which create a greater threat to conventional care – and patients' welfare – than do spurious arguments of putative benefits from absurd dilutions".

Editor of *Lancet* rightly tells,

Surely the time has passed for selective analyses, biased reports, or further investment in research

Chapter fifty six: Research on homeopathy

251

> to perpetuate the homoeopathy versus allopathy debate. Now doctors need to be bold and honest with their patients about homoeopathy's lack of benefit, and with themselves about the failings of modern medicine to address patients' needs for personalised care. (Editorial, 2005).

When Hahnemann principles of homeopathy are not according to principles of basic medical science and basic biological science, then any clinical trial or research study should not show any therapeutic effect of homeopathic remedy But there are many research papers that show therapeutic effects of homeopathic compounds. Some trials also mention greater than placebo effects by homeopathic remedies. Now there is a very important question. When a therapeutic system is against basic medical science, then how can it show a therapeutic effect which is greater than placebo? Answer is very simple. These trials have serious methodological flaws, weaknesses in study design and reporting, small sample size, and selection bias. Bias in the conduct and reporting of trials is also an explanation. Usually, results of trials were not replicated. They didn't include enough participants to have meaningful results, or the researchers failed to limit bias and control for confounding factors. Quality of the evidence was low or unclear. Due to these limitations, such studies are not reliable for making conclusions in favor of homeopathy.

In fact the high-quality studies did not find that homeopathy performed better than a placebo for a range of health conditions, including asthma, anxiety, chronic fatigue syndrome, colds, and ulcers. Better quality trials have become available, the evidence for efficacy of homeopathy preparations has diminished.

Systematic reviews and meta-analysis of clinical trials and scientific principles have proved that homeopathic remedies are not therapeutically effective. They are no better than placebo. This homeopathy is also responsible for the increase of morbidity and mortality of thousands of patients who ignore treatment of modern medical science. It's a good time to decide to stop investing government research funding in this therapy. The treatment doesn't work, and people should stop wasting their time, money, and energy on this useless system of therapy. People's acceptance of any therapeutic system is not related to its effectiveness. Spontaneous recovery of many diseases gives false impressions of the utility of different therapeutic systems. Only scientific analysis, animal studies, and clinical trials explain the truth. On such a basis, we have known that homeopathy is a pseudo, illogical, unscientific, and ineffective system of treatment.

References

Aabel, S. (2000). No beneficial effect of isopathic prophylactic treatment for birch pollen allergy during a low-pollen season: A double-blind, placebo-controlled clinical trial of homeopathic Betula 30c. *British Homoeopathic Journal, 89*(4), 169–173. doi: 10.1054/homp.1999.0440.

Agence France-Presse in Paris (2019, July 10). France to stop reimbursing patients for homeopathy | France. *The Guardian*. Retrieved from·https://www.theguardian.com/world/2019/jul/10/france-to-stop-reimbursing-patients-for-homeopathic-treatment

Baum, M., & Ernst, E. (2009). Should we maintain an open mind about homeopathy? *American Journal of Medicine, 122*(11), 973–974. doi: 10.1016/j.amjmed.2009.03.038.

Belluz, J. (2016, November 18). The US government is finally telling people that homeopathy is a sham. *Vox News*. Retrieved from https://www.vox.com/2016/11/18/13676834/ftc-homeopathy-crackdown-regulation

Cucherat, M., Haugh, M. C., Gooch, M., & Boissel, J. P. (2000). Evidence of clinical efficacy of homeopathy. A meta-analysis of clinical trials. HMRAG. Homeopathic medicines research advisory group. *European Journal of Clinical Pharmacology, 56*(1), 27–33. doi: 10.1007/s002280050716.

Davey, M. (2015, March 11). Homeopathy not effective for treating any condition – Australian report finds. *The Guardian*. Retrieved from https://www.theguardian.com/lifeandstyle/2015/mar/11/homeopathy-not-effective-for-treating-any-condition-australian-report-finds

Dearden, L. (2017, February 7). The Russian Academy of Sciences says homeopathy is dangerous pseudoscience that does not work. *The Independent*. Retrieved from https://www.independent.co.uk/news/world/europe/russia-academy-of-sciences-homeopathy-treaments-pseudoscience-does-not-work-par-magic-a7566406.html

EASAC (2017, September 20). *The European Academies' Science Advisory Council reports regarding use of homeopathic products*. Retrieved from https://easac.eu/publications/details/homeopathic-products-and-practices/

Editorial (2005). The end of homoeopathy. *The Lancet, 366*(9487), 690.

Ernst, E. (2002). A systematic review of systematic reviews of homeopathy. *British Journal of Clinical Pharmacology, 54*(6), 577–582. doi: 10.1046/j.1365-2125.2002.01699.x.

Güell, O. (2018, November 14). Spain moves to ban pseudo-therapies from universities and health centers. *EL PAÍS*. English version by Melissa Kitson. Retrieved from https://english.elpais.com/author/melissa-kitson/

Jonas, W. B., Anderson, R. L., Crawford, C., & Lyons, J. S. (2001). A systematic review of the quality of homeopathic clinical trials. *BMC Complementary Medicine and Therapies, 1*, 12. doi: 10.1186/1472-6882-1-12.

Kleijnen, J., Knipschild, P., & Riet, G. T. (1991). Clinical trials of homoeopathy. *British Medical Journal, 302*(6772), 316–323. doi: 10.1136/bmj.302.6772.316.

Linde, K., Clausius, N., Ramirez, G., Melchart, D., Eitel, F., Hedges, L. V., & Jonas, W. B. (1997). Are the clinical effects of homeopathy placebo effects? A meta-analysis of placebo-controlled trials. *The Lancet, 350*(9081), 834–843. doi: 10.1016/s0140-6736(97)02293-9.

Chapter fifty six: Research on homeopathy 253

Litvinova, D. (2017, February 9). Russian scientists rally against the rise of homeopathic pseudo-Medicine. *The Moscow Times*. Retrieved from https://www.themoscowtimes.com/2017/02/09/the-magic-potion-scientists-condemn-homeopathy-but-russians-are-not-convinced-a57088

Mathie, R. T., Lloyd, S. M., & Legg, L. A. et al. (2014). Randomised placebo-controlled trials of individualised homeopathic treatment: Systematic review and meta-analysis. *Systematic Reviews, 3*, 142. doi: 10.1186/2046-4053-3-142.

Ramesh, S. (2020, March 11). Forget coronavirus, homoeopathy can't cure anything. It's a placebo, at best. *The Print*. Retrieved from https://theprint.in/science/forget-coronavirus-homoeopathy-cant-cure-anything-its-a-placebo-at-best/363174/

Shaddel, F., Ghazirad, M., & Bryant, M. (2014). What is the best available evidence for using homeopathy in patients with intellectual disabilities? *Iranian Journal of Pediatrics, 24*(4), 339–344.

Shang, A., Müntener, K. H., Nartey, L., Jüni, P., Dörig, S., Sterne, J. A. C., Pewsner, D., & Egger, M. (2005). Are the clinical effects of homoeopathy placebo effects? Comparative study of placebo-controlled trials of homoeopathy and allopathy. *The Lancet, 366*(9487), 726–732. doi: 10.1016/S0140-6736(05)67177-2.

Smith, K. (2012). Homeopathy is unscientific and unethical. *Bioethics, 26*(9), 508–512. https://doi.org/10.1111/j.1467-8519.2011.0195.x.

Subhranil, S., & Munmun, K. (2013). Homeopathic treatment of headaches and migraine: A meta-analysis of the randomized controlled trials. *Asian Journal of Pharmaceutical and Clinical Research, 6*(7), 194–199. Systematic review registration number: CRD42013004714; date 29 May 2013

The National Association of Statutory Health Insurance Physicians (NASHIP) (2019, July 11). German health insurers urged to end homeopathy refunds | News. *DW*. Retrieved from https://www.dw.com/en/german-health-insurers-urged-to-end-homeopathy-refunds/a-49546319

UK Science and Technology Committee (2010, February 22). British House and Technology Committee Report on homeopathy. Retrieved from https://publications.parliament.uk/pa/cm200910/cmselect/cmsctech/45/4502.htm

Vithoulkas, G. (2017). Serious mistakes in meta-analysis of homeopathic research. *Journal of Medicine and Life, 10*(1), 47–49.

chapter fifty seven

Conclusion

Basic concept of this book: homeopathy – an illusion of effectiveness: fifty seven

Principles of homeopathy are wrong and Hahnemann framed these rules of homeopathy on wrong foundations that are against principles of basic medical science. Homeopathy has no therapeutic utility. It is an illusion of effectiveness only.

Explanation

When we conclude that all principles of homeopathy are wrong and Hahnemann framed these rules of homeopathy on wrong foundations that are against principles of basic medical science, then what is the logic behind analyzing these clinical trials related to homeopathic remedies.

When basic principles of homeopathy are wrong, then it is not possible that any clinical trial should show a positive effect of any homeopathic remedy. If a clinical trial or study shows effectiveness of homeopathic substance, it only indicates defect in methodology of trial or bias to manipulate the result. If we make plans to study to show the effectiveness of homeopathic remedies, it means we are creating doubts on principles of basic medical and biological science and it is not justice to those scientists who have contributed to the development of available medical knowledge.

Drug is a substance or product that is used or intended to be used to modify or explore the physiological system or the pathological state for the benefit of the recipient. This is the definition of drug, as explained by WHO. Therapeutic application of drug requires detailed knowledge of it.

Knowledge regarding absorption, drug transport, plasma concentration, equivalence, bioavailability, distribution, binding of drug in tissues, plasma protein binding, metabolism, site of metabolism, excretion, clearance, plasma half-life, dose-response curve, dosing schedule, duration of action, site of drug action, mechanism of drug action, safety of drug, therapeutic index, adverse drug effect, drug interaction, structure-activity relationship, preclinical animal study, and different phases of clinical trials are required to use a substance as a drug for patients.

DOI: 10.1201/9781003228622-57

Homeopathic remedies do not contain active gradients due to higher dilutions. There is no substance in homeopathic preparation. Being a drug, there should be a substance. In the absence of a single molecule of a substance, homeopathic remedy cannot be named as a drug.

Before clinical trials of a drug, preclinical animal study is required. Preliminary pharmacodynamic screening in animals is a must for further study. The effects of different doses are investigated in mice or other animals and the profile of activity is studied. The compound is administered intravenously to intact animals such as dogs or cats to see the effect on different physiological systems. The investigation is extended to isolated tissues, e.g., guinea pig ileum and rat uterus. If a compound has prominent activity in preliminary screening, then it is further investigated in several species of animals in various models of diseases.

After preliminary pharmacological study in animals, toxicity studies are performed in animals with specific compounds intended to be used in clinical trials. Acute toxicity, subacute toxicity, chronic toxicity, and effect on reproduction, mutagenicity, and carcinogenicity are evaluated. When a compound is cleared from toxicological studies, pharmacokinetic studies are performed in various species of animals such as rats, dogs, and monkeys to know regarding absorption, drug transport, plasma concentration, bioavailability, distribution, binding of drug in tissues, plasma protein binding, metabolism, excretion, clearance, and plasma half-life.

After animal study, clinical trials or studies in human beings are performed. It includes pharmacokinetic studies, safety, and efficacy of drugs. There are four phases of clinical trials. In phase 1 of clinical trials, investigation of safety is the main concern. The findings of pharmacokinetic processes, obtained in animal studies, are confirmed in human beings. It is non-blind. Thirty to fifty healthy volunteers or volunteer patients are taken in this study. In phase 2 of clinical trials, 50–300 patients as subjects are taken. Efficacy is the main concern in this study. It is double blind; dose range and comparison with placebo are carried out. Phase 2 trials can also be considered a part of formal therapeutic trials.

Phase 3 clinical trial is a trial of therapeutic confirmation and the aim of study is to confirm finding of phase 2 on a large scale. Efficacy and safety are the main concerns. Two hundred fifty to one thousand patients are taken in the study. It is double blind study. Comparison with existing standard drugs is also performed. After a successful phase 3 trial, the drug is marketed after necessary permission from the regulatory authorities. Phase 4 of the clinical trial is actually post-marketing surveillance. In this phase, 2500 to 10,000 patients are taken for study. To observe adverse drug effects, comparison with existing drugs and studies in special groups (elderly people, children, pregnant ladies) are the main targets of study in this phase.

Chapter fifty seven: Conclusion 257

If homeopathic remedies do not contain any active gradient, then there is no use of doing any clinical trial. It is just a waste of time and money. If homeopathic remedies have activity on the biological system, then animal study should be necessary before clinical trials. Without such studies, clinical trials cannot be allowed. But scientists are allowed to do clinical trials without animal study; however, it is absolutely wrong. Without animal study, nobody should be allowed to do clinical trials.

Similarly, without doing phase 1 of clinical trial in human beings, permission for doing formal therapeutic trials should not be granted. But it is unfortunate that without doing animal study and phase 1 clinical trials, permission for formal therapeutic trials is being given by regulating authorities.

Please stop trials and study in relation to homeopathic remedies. It can be explained by the following example. A patient has died in hospital. His brain and heart stopped functioning. His body started deteriorating. Foul smell is there. After 24 hours of his death, physicians are discussing how to maintain the blood pressure of that dead patient. They are trying to give blood and saline to him. Nurse is forcefully opening the mouth of the dead body and forcefully inserting food. They are not ready to accept the fact that the patient has died. Nobody is ready for the cremation or burial of that dead patient. This is the best example to show the prevalence of homeopathy in the world. Actually what is happening,

> Alternative medicine also distinguishes itself by an ideology that largely ignores biological mechanisms, often disparages modern science, and relies on what are purported to be ancient practices and natural remedies (more potent and less toxic than conventional medicine). Accordingly, herbs or mixtures of herbs are considered superior to the active compounds isolated in the laboratory. And healing methods such as homeopathy and therapeutic touch are fervently promoted despite not only the lack of good clinical evidence of effectiveness, but the presence of a rationale that violates fundamental scientific laws. (Angell & Kassirer, 1998)

To prevent academic pollution and reach the right conclusion, principles of modern medical science should be applied to analyze alternative therapies also. Alternative treatment should be subjected to the same scientific testing as required for conventional treatment.

258   *Homeopathy*

Angell and Kassirer rightly said,

> It is time for the scientific community to stop giving alternative medicine a free ride. There cannot be two kinds of medicine, a conventional and alternative. There is only medicine that has been adequately tested and medicine that has not, medicine that works and medicine that may or may not work. Once a treatment has been tested rigorously, it no longer matters whether it was considered alternative at the outset. If it is found to be reasonably safe and effective, it will be accepted. But assertions, speculation, and testimonials do not substitute for evidence.(Angell & Kassirer, 1998)

Nowadays, the concept of old allopathy has been totally changed. Today developed medical science is based on scientific study, experiments, and controlled observations. Purgation, blood removal, and the concept of plethora are not accepted today. Electrolytes and fluid are administered in dehydrated conditions and blood is also administered when required. Knowledge of different branches of science is being used in the medical field. New advanced methods of investigation are being used today. Morbidity and mortality are also reducing day by day. Today we have vast knowledge.

Acceptance of homeopathy indicates our ignorance, lack of knowledge, unscientific approach, and inability to understand science. Prevalence of homeopathy in 2022 AD is against society, humanity, and intelligence. Societies and nations are losing money, time, and lives by supporting homeopathy.

The aim of this work was to analyze mistakes done by Hahnemann. Now we know that Hahnemann made many mistakes. Now there is also no doubt that homeopathy has no therapeutic effect. Whatever beneficial effect obtained by homeopathic drugs is actually a placebo effect. We have also discussed that placebo therapeutic effect is a psychological effect and such effect can be obtained by inert substances also.

At one time, homeopathy protected the public from ill effects of old allopathic treatment. At present, homeopathy is misleading the public and increasing morbidity and mortality because it is interfering in the application of modern medical science.That's why,

Homeopathy should be discarded.
Homeopathy should be banned.
Homeopathy has no curative ability.

Chapter fifty seven: Conclusion   *259*

Homeopathy has no therapeutic utility.
It is an illusion of effectiveness only.

Reference

Angell, M., & Kassirer, J. P. (1998). Alternative medicine – The risks of untested
and unregulated remedies. *The New England Journal of Medicine, 339*(12),
839–841 https://doi.org/10.1056/nejm199809173391210.

Index

A

Aabel, S., 241
Abdominal pain, 24
Accepted failure, Hahnemann, 227–237
Acidosis, 72
Acute disease, 46, 145–148, 224; *see also*
    Chronic disease
  causes of, 149
  into chronic diseases, 173–174, 223
  complications, 79
  prognostic, 55
Acute mercury poisoning, 52
Acute varicella (chickenpox), 119
Agence France-Presse in Paris, 248
AIDS, 13, 20–21, 81, 104–105, 107, 145, 227
Allopathic drugs, 93, 173, 175–177
  modifying acute into chronic
    diseases, 174
  in sexually transmitted disease, 182
  suppressing gonorrhea in male,
    179–180
  toxicity of, 187
Allopathy, xv, 258
  Ayurveda and Unani, 25
  criticism of, 9–11
  damaging effect of, 236
  principles of, 10
  use of chemicals, 176
Alopecia areata, 119
Amitriptyline, 26
Amoxicillin, 20
Ampicillin, 26
Angell, M., 258
Angina, 17
Antacids, 26
Antibiotics, 20–21, 26, 77–78, 110, 155, 174

Antidepressant drugs, 26
Antigen
  administered in animal, 30
  antibody, 29
  cox virus and smallpox virus, 30
  delayed hypersensitivity
    reactions, 215
  stimulus, 102–103
  structure, 31, 106
Antigen-antibody, 102–105
  complexes, 103–105
  reaction, 102–104
Antihypertensive drugs, 26
Antileprosy drugs, 26
Antimony, 176
Antipsoric medicine/drugs, 157, 234;
    see also Medicine
Antipsychotic drugs, 26
Antitubercular drugs, 26
Antituberculosis chemotherapy, 110;
    see also Tuberculosis
Arsenic, 67
  compound, 159, 182
  dilutions of, 159
  elementary, 68
  homeopathic use in dysentery, 76
  metallic, 68
  in syphilis, 155, 158, 176, 187
  toxicities/poisoning, 183–185
Artificial diseases, 1, 27, 45, 48
Asthma, 17
  allergic, 209–210
  manifested clinically, 209
  manifested physiologically, 209
  and reappearance of skin lesions, 89
  and ulceration of lungs, 33, 89
Ayurveda, 9–10, 25, 37, 110–111, 230

262 Index

B

Bacillary dysentery, 20
Bacillus typhosus, 51, 53
Back pain, 118
Bacteria (microbial agents), 19
    antibiotics/chemotherapeutic drugs,
        20–21, 77, 110, 114
    Calymmatobacterium granulomatis, 167
    diseases/infection, 24, 79–80, 93,
        102–103, 179, 215
    external, 24
    gonorrhea, 170
    as harmless, 135–140
    inoculation in animals, 21
    invasion, 215
    isolation, 102, 165
    mercury effect on, 53
    Neisseria gonorrhoeae, 170
    not accepted by homeopathy, 76
    Salmonella, 20
    sterilization, 77
    transmission, 21–22
    tuberculosis, 109
Baum, M., 241–242
Belladonna, 63–66
Belluz, J., 248–249
Biases, 240, 242, 245–246, 251, 255
Bismuth, 155, 176, 182, 185
Bloodletting, 9–10, 71
Body parts, 133–134
Bright's disease, 113–114, 127–128, 182, 184
Buzyn, A., 248

C

Calymmatobacterium granulomatis, 20, 167
Camphor, 72; *see also* Cholera
Cancer/carcinomas, 17, 33, 35, 76–77, 80,
        120, 134, 140, 168, 208, 229
    of breast, 232
    of the lips and face, 89
    removal of, 90
    spread of, 89
    therapy, 120
    treatment, 35, 120
Cannon, W. B., 47
Cennino, 69
Chancre
    burning by caustics, 89
    chancroid and, 173–174
    external, 157

    and figwart, 203, 219
    general chancre disease, 147
    internal syphilis, 88
    painless, 158
    primary, 150, 152–153, 165–166
    soft, 153
    venereal, 33, 163, 201
Chancroid
    chancre and, 152, 173–174
    defined, 168
    gonorrhea and, 176
    Haemophilus ducreyi, 20, 152
    sexually transmitted diseases, 149
    systemic symptoms, 153
    ulcers of, 153
Chickenpox, 79–80, 104, 116, 119
Chlamydia, 23, 165, 168
Chlamydia trachomatis, 167
Chloramphenicol, 20
Chlorpromazine, 26
Cholera, 20, 76, 80, 100, 115, 227, 236
    medicine, 73
    spread prevention, 21
    treatment of, 71–73, 78
Chronic diseases, 117, 123, 145–148, 207,
        221–224; *see also* Acute disease
    acute diseases into, 174
    advanced, 232
    causes of, 33–34, 149, 199
    natural, 83
    older, 79
    recovery, 234
    sinful thoughts and acts, 75
    suppressing other chronic
        disease, 127
    suppression of eruption and
        itch, 204
    treatment of, 234–235
Chronic mercury poisoning, 52
Cinchona bark, 1–2, 144
Ciprofloxacin, 26
Clinical trials, 239, 244–245, 249, 251,
        255–257
Clostridium oedematiens, 138
Clostridium septicum, 138
Clostridium tetani, 20
Clostridium welchii, 138
Colloids, 68–69
Condyloma acuminata, 165–166, 168;
        see also Genital wart
Condylomata, 89, 150, 166
Confusion, 52, 63, 219–220

Index 263

Cowpox
  inoculation, 31, 102, 106
  symptomatology of, 105
  virus, 106
Cox virus, 30
Cucherat, M., 243
Curative power of medicine, 39–43
Cures
  means removal of symptoms, 17
  mechanism of, 25–27

D

Davey, M., 242
Deadening, 5
Dearden, L., 247–248
Degenerative neurological diseases, 17
Dehydration, 72, 80, 236
Delirium, 92–93, 133
Dengue, 215–216
Depression, 2, 6, 26, 60, 102
Dermatophytosis, 118
Diabetes, 17, 35, 77–78, 106, 113–114, 134, 140,
      200, 228–229
Diagnosis
  clinical, 201
  differential, 171, 176
  of disease, 13
  Donovan bodies, 167
  etiological agents, 149
  of infective diseases, 102
  of malaria, 3
  role of pathological investigations in,
      23–24
  of viral disease, 30
Diarrhoea, 71, 114, 117, 143, 155, 185, 203, 216
Dilution, 1, 97, 158, 239, 250, 256
  arsenic, 159
  camphor, 72
  increase in potency due to, 5–7, 42
  mercuric chloride, 51
  trituration/succussion, 40, 67–68, 95
Diseases; see also Chronic diseases
  acute, 46
  artificial, 1, 27, 45, 48
  bacteria (microbial agents), 24, 79–80, 93,
      102–103, 179, 215
  diagnosis of, 13, 15
  etiology of, 13
  external factors for, 19–22
  infectious, 29
  interaction of, 29–31

knowledge regarding, 13–14
nomenclature of, 15
protection from another disease,
      113–116
venereal, 163, 165–171, 207
Displacement of pathological symptoms,
      45–50
Dissimilar diseases, 113
  suffering with two, 101–107
Disturbed psyche, 77
Dose, 171, 256
  of arsenic, 159
  effective, 1
  of homeopathic drug, 49, 93, 224
  infective, 115
  infinitesimal, 63
  of mercury compound, 156
  moderate, 40
  repetition of, 221–225
  response curve, 42, 255
  smallness of, 64
  strong and opposite symptoms, 41
Dynamization, 95–97, 156
Dysentery, treatment, 9

E

Epilepsy, 17, 29, 33, 48, 80, 200
  and exanthema, 213–217
  leptazol, 48
Ergotism, 196–197
Ernst, E., 240–241
Erysipelas, 120, 137–138, 196, 200, 215–216
Erythromycins, 26
Ethanol
  concentration of blood, 6
  physiological effects of, 6
Euphoria, 6, 56
European Academies' Science Advisory
      Council (EASAC), 245–246
Exanthema, 213–217
Exorcism, 91

F

Fever, 99–100
  accompanying cowpox, 102
  associated with self-limited
      infections, 118
  cat scratch, 217
  causes of, 23
  diagnosis, 23

epidemic, 101, 144
gastric, 234
inflammatory, 123
malarial, 2
paroxysm of, 3
in pneumocystis carinii
pneumonia, 114
rheumatic, 217
scarlet, 63–66, 215–216, 236
suppression of itch, 215
symptoms of, 3
tinea capitis, 208
typhoid, 20, 78, 117, 215, 227
yellow, 100, 217
Fig warts, 147, 163, 171, 179–186, 201,
203, 219
Fistula in ano, 131–132
Fungicide, 56
Fungi/fungus, 20–21, 33, 56, 196, 208–209

G

Generalization, 1, 5, 31, 53, 56, 88,
131–132, 197
Genital herpes, 165, 170
Genital wart, 165, 168–169, 171
Gold, 67–69
Gonorrhoea/gonorrhea, 84, 132, 153, 170
discharge suppressed by allopathic
injection, 163–164
fig-wart diseases and, 179–186
genital warts, 171, 180
Neisseria gonorrhoeae, 170
sexually transmitted diseases,
149, 165
symptom of, 166
syphilis diagnosed as, 176
types, 179
Gottheil, E. S., 188
Granuloma inguinale, 20, 131, 149,
165–168, 176
Grinding, 67–69
Güell, O., 246–247
Gumma/gummata, 128, 150, 188

H

Haemophilus ducreyi, 20, 152–153
Haemophilus influenzae, 215
Hemiplegia, 134
Hemorrhoids, 171, 200
Herpes simplex, 119; *see also* Warts

Herpes zoster, 103, 119
Hippocrates, xiii
Homeostasis, 47
Hunter, John, 173
Hydrophobia, 135, 227
Hyperpyrexia, 99
Hypertension, 17, 35
Hypothyroidism, 11

I

Imipramine, 26
Immunity
and antigen antibody reaction, 29,
102, 104
cellular, 104
hypersensitivity reaction, 103
protective role in polio and viral
infections, 103
to reinfection, 30
role in disease development, 102
to scarlet fever, 64, 66
viral and bacterial diseases, 24
Immunization, 29
Incubation period, 115
Infectious diseases, 29; *see also* Diseases
Injection, 99–100
allopathic, 76, 163, 175, 177
intramuscular, 182
of mercury or bismuth, 182
of soluble mercurial salts, 155
therapeutic effect of, 156
Interferons, 115
cellular glycoprotein, 106
described, 106–107
produced by acute viral infection, 31
protein, 30
protozoal infection developing, 107
synthesis, 107
Internal psora, 88, 197, 200, 203–205; *see also*
Psora
Investigations, rejection of, 23–24
Iodine, use in hypothyroidism, 11
Itch
dry, 213
exaltation of, 56
internal, 196
miasma of, 201
psora, 147, 163
suppression of, 203–205, 207–210,
213–215, 217, 220
vesicles, 202

Index

265

J

Johnson, V. E., 157
Jonas, W. B., 249

K

Kassirer, J. P., 258
Kent, J. T., 19, 42–43, 109–110, 113–115, 127,
 131, 133–134, 135–139, 152, 158,
 180–183, 187, 191–192, 195–196
Kleijnen, J., 245

L

Lancet, 250
Lavaditi, 185
Legionella, 20
Leprosy
 bacteria behind, 137
 drugs, 26
 homeopathy denying bacteria
  behind, 77
 Mycobacterium leprae, 20
 St. Anthony's fire and, 195–198
Leptazol, 48
Leptospira, 20
Linde, K., 244–245
Lithium, plasma concentration of, 7
Litvinova, D., 247–248
Lobar pneumonia, 228
Lymphogranuloma venereum, 149, 165–167

M

Malaria/malarial
 cinchona use in, 51
 in diabetes patient, 106
 diagnosis, 3
 drugs, 51, 75
 as not fatal disease, 227
 parasites, 23, 75
 paroxysm, 1–2
 quinine use in, 11
 relapse of, 2–3
 spread of, 21–22
 spread prevention, 21–22
 transmission of, 3, 75
 treatment, 9, 75
Mania, 7, 33, 59–60, 80, 92, 140, 197, 200
Masters, W. H., 157
Mathie, R. T., 244

Measles, 100, 116, 215–216
 absence of rashes in, 104
 in an epidemic, 101
 case fatality rates, 228
 chances of spontaneous recovery, 236
 immunization, 103
 live attenuated virus, 106
 of the lung, 102
 prevalence of, 31
 smallpox and, 106
Medical science, 111, 120, 237
 advanced, 144
 basic, 251, 255
 criticizing, 9, 11
 development, 75, 91, 101
 modern, 11, 14, 37, 73, 91, 251, 257–258
Medicine
 alternative, 248, 257–258
 curative power of, 39–43
 dose and, 221–225
 employed in cholera, 73
 homeopathic, 95
 pathogenic effect, 39
 requisite, 23
Melampus, 59
Meningitis, 20
Mercuric chloride, 5
 syphilis and, 51–53
Mercuric oxide, 5
Mercury, 188
 acute mercury poisoning, 52
 chronic mercury poisoning, 52
 compounds, 156, 184–185
 concentration/concentrated, 53, 67, 176,
  183
 dilution/trituration of, 67–68
 elemental, 5
 proto iodide of, 155
 salts of, 5, 52
 toxicity/poisoning, 52, 93, 183
 trituration of, 5–6
 use in syphilis, 51, 176, 187
Meta-analysis, 240, 243–245, 249, 251
Methylmercury, 6
Miasm
 acute, 179
 chronic, 83, 85, 147–149, 163, 179
 of psora, 202
 sycosis, 166, 168, 171
 syphilitic, 165, 166
Microorganism, 140
Morphine, 56, 136

Moxa, 71, 144
Mumps, 30–31, 100, 102, 115–116, 217;
    see also Measles
Munmun, K., 245
Mycobacterium leprae, 20
Mycobacterium tuberculosis, 20
Myocardial infarction, 17

N

National Association of Statutory
        Health Insurance Physicians
        (NASHIP), 248
National Health and Medical
        Research Council (NHMRC)
        Australia, 242
Natural disease, 39, 47–49, 174
Neisseria gonorrhoeae, 170
Neoarsphenamine, 159
Nephritic syndrome, 52, 127–128
Nomenclature of diseases, 15

O

Old school of medicine, 143–144
Opium, effect of, 55–56
Organon of Medicine (Hahnemann), 25
Organs of the body, *see* Body parts
Oxygenation, 139

P

Parasiticide, 56
Paroxysm
    of fever with chill, 3
    malaria, 1–2
Pathogenesis, 14
    of an exanthem, 215
    defined, 21
    of disease, 11, 207
    of psora, 199–202
    of the spread of cancer, 89
    symptomatology, 13
    T. pallidum, 53
Pathological investigations
    rejection of, 23–24
    role in diagnosis, 23–24
Pathological symptoms
    displacement of, 45–50
Penicillin, 53, 159, 176, 216
Peptic ulcer, 17
Persistent virus infections, 30

Pharmacodynamic, 11, 42, 111, 183, 230, 256
Pharmacokinetic, 11, 42–43, 111, 122, 183,
        230, 256
Pityriasis rosea, 119
Platinum, 67–68
Pneumonia, 20
Potency, 1, 97, 156, 234
    2c, 96
    3c, 96
    dilution role in, 5–7, 67
    drug therapeutic, 26, 95
    LM 30, 96
    thirtieth (30th), 7, 39–40, 42, 48–49, 76,
        156
    trituration in, 5, 67
Proctitis, 117
Proteus, 59
Protozoa, 21
Psora, 33, 75–78
    development of, 79–81, 202
    evolution, 195
    internal, 88, 197, 200, 203–205
    manifestations, 83–84, 157
    pathogenesis of, 199–202
    and spiritualism, 191–193
    suppressed by wrong treatment, 84
    suppression of, 175, 177
Psychiatric symptoms, 91–93
Ptomaine, 137–138

Q

Quinine
    analgesic and antipyretic action, 2
    use in malaria, 11

R

Rabies, 13, 81, 100, 117, 135, 227
Ramesh, S., 242–243
Respiratory tract infections, 20, 26
Rickettsias, 23
Rigors or chills, 2
Ringworm, 29, 84, 208
Ross, Ronald, 3, 75

S

Salivation, 185
Salmonella, 20
Sazerac, 185

Index

267

Scarlet fever, 63–66, 215–216, 236; *see also* Fever
Schizophrenia, 26
Septicaemia, 137
Septran, 20
Sexually transmitted diseases, 24, 149, 165, 171, 176–177, 199, 229
Shaddel, F., 245
Shang, A., 240, 250
Shingles, *see* Herpes zoster
Silver, 5, 11, 51–52, 67–68, 184
Skin diseases, 76, 83–85, 118
Slow virus infections, 30
Smallpox
    caused by variola virus, 105
    causing swelling, 31
    inoculation of, 101
    management of, 236
    skin lesions, 104
    vaccines/vaccination, 100, 102, 105–106
    virus, 30, 106, 140
Smith, K., 239–240
Spirochetes, 20
St. Anthony's Fire, 195–198
Staphylococcal scalded skin syndrome (SSSS), 118
Staphylococcus aureus, 118
Subhranil, S., 245
Succussion, 96, 223
    and trituration, 40, 67
Sulfamethoxazole, 26
Sulfur, 11, 55–56, 184, 203, 220
Suppressed manifestations, 158, 187–189
Sycosis, 163–164, 179, 181
    chronic disease, 147
    miasm, 166, 168, 171
    syphilis and, 76, 147, 164, 193, 197, 199, 207, 227
    treatment, 164
Sycosis miasm, 166, 168, 171
Syphilis, 20, 33, 145, 171, 229
    Bright's disease and, 127–128
    causes termination of life, 149–153
    mercuric chloride and, 51–53
    suppressed, 84, 187
    sycosis and, 76, 147, 164, 193, 197, 199, 207, 227
    symptomatology, 51–52
    treatment, 35, 52, 128, 150, 155–160, 164, 176, 185, 187–188

Treponema pallidum, 30
    wrong generalization, 88
Systematic reviews, 240–243, 251

T

Tetanus, 20
Therapeutic effectiveness, 117–123
Thioridazine, 26
Tinea capitis, 200, 202, 207–210, 219
Trachoma, 20
Trephine, 71
Treponema pallidum, 20, 52–53, 150, 158–159
Treponema pertenue, 20
Trimethoprim, 26
Trituration, 97
    dilution and, 67–68, 95
    of mercury, 5–6, 67
    and succussion, 40, 67
Tuberculosis, 20, 77, 109–111, 196
    bacteria in, 137
    fistula in ano, 131
    genital, 168
    mortality, 110
    mycobacterium, 104, 109–110
    patients, 104
    pulmonary, 101, 105
    symptomatology/symptoms of, 26, 114
    treatment, 35, 99, 110
Typhoid, 22, 26, 76–77
    cure/treatment, 227, 236
    fever, 20, 78, 117, 215
    infections, 20, 78, 116

U

UK Science and Technology Committee, 243–244
Unani, 25
Urinary tract infections, 20

V

Vaccination, 99–100
    smallpox coming on after, 102, 105–106
Venereal diseases, 163, 165–171, 207
Venesections, 11, 71, 123
Veratrum, 59–60
Vibrio cholerae, 72
Viral diseases, 24, 80, 107

268 *Index*

Vital force, 45, 48, 136, 146–147, 202, 222
  curative power of, 47
  drug-induced effect, 49
  ineradicable, 163
  insufficient, 148
  organic, 88
  preserving, 89
  self acting (automatic), 46
Vithoulkas, G., 249–250

W

Warts
  antibodies, 169
  defined, 119
  due to sycosis, 164
  fig, 147, 163, 171, 179–186, 201, 203, 219
  genital, 165, 168–169, 171
  and localized treatment, 87–90
  treatment, 117, 169
Weil's disease, 20
Welch, William, 160

Y

Yaws, 20